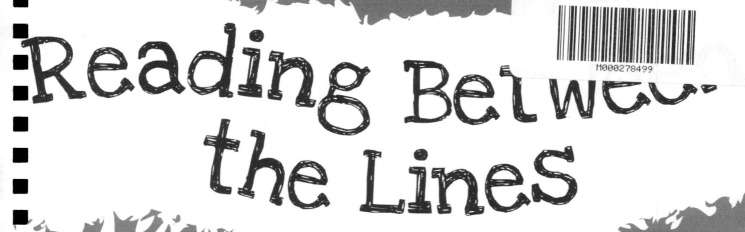

Reading Between the Lines

Teaching Children to Understand Inference

Catherine Delamain & Jill Spring

Speechmark

First published in 2014 by

Speechmark Publishing Ltd

St Mark's House, Shepherdess Walk, London N1 7BQ, United Kingdom

www.speechmark.net

Reprinted 2015

002-5898 Printed in the United Kingdom by CMP (uk) Ltd

British Library Cataloguing in Publication Data
A catalogue record for this book is available from the British Library.

ISBN: 978 0 86388 969 1

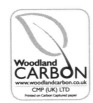

CONTENTS

PREFACE

Language is a process of free creation; its laws and principles are fixed, but the manner in which the principles of generation are used is free and infinitely varied. Even the interpretation and use of words involves a process of free creation Paul Tillich

The ability to draw inference is a vital part of understanding language. It is needed for grasping subtleties, innuendos, humour, emotions, contrasts and comparisons. Inference is defined as making deductions or coming to conclusions based on the given facts, world knowledge and reasoning. It is also often referred to as understanding things that are not spelt out in so many words. It is important that children are helped where necessary to acquire this essential skill. Many children in mainstream classes have problems in 'getting the main idea', while children with language and communication needs are particularly likely to find it difficult.

The authors of this book have many years' experience of collaborative working with teachers in a range of educational settings, and are aware of the time constraints faced by staff. Teachers and teaching assistants do not have the time to trawl through the contents of the school library to find appropriate texts, and there is very little available in the way of published material. *Reading Between the Lines* aims to fill this gap.

This book contains 300 short texts providing practice in drawing inference. It is designed for children in Key Stage 2, who will range in age from 7 to 11 years, and can be used with both readers and non-readers. The authors hope it will prove a useful tool in developing language comprehension in its fullest sense.

Reading Between the Lines offers:

- Graded texts covering the 10 main categories of inference

- Clear instructions and hints on use

- A template for optional record keeping

INTRODUCTION

> **Man's ultimate concern must be expressed symbolically, because symbolic language alone is able to express the ultimate.** Paul Tillich

The National Curriculum pays much attention to language enrichment and the development of both spoken and written language. There is increasing emphasis on the comprehension of written texts, but the development of inferential skills is assumed rather than directly addressed.

Development of inference

By the age of about seven the typically developing child will be able to read a straightforward text supported by pictures, and understand what it is about. For example:

Johnny kicked the ball.

The child can see what is happening and link it to the words he has read.

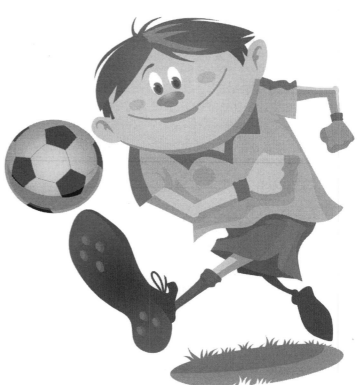

The next step is a bit more difficult. This is where the child needs to be able to see beyond the words on the page and involves understanding what they have read, and at the same time using their knowledge of the world and grasp of the key elements in the story to draw inference from unstated information.

For example:

When Mr Jones opened the letter, his life changed for ever.

The child can read the words and tell from the picture that Mr Jones is pleased about something. However, the child needs their 'world knowledge' to think what that might be, such as a lottery or betting win, a legacy or a sudden cash windfall.

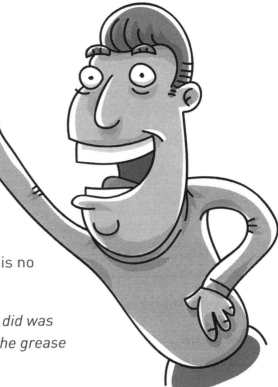

The hardest type of inference occurs when there is no visual support. For example:

When Ted came home from work, the first thing he did was drop his overalls in the washing basket and scrub the grease off his hands.

What kind of job did Ted do?

The child needs to work out that Ted was dirty, and needs to use world knowledge to guess what kind of job he might do.

The child who relies solely on direct information given in the text or in pictures will find it increasingly difficult to make sense of more complex text. This is particularly true in the case of fiction, where inference is needed to understand depth of meaning, including feelings, mood, atmosphere and tension.

Many children learn to decode text competently but fail to develop inferencing skills. This limits their ability to identify the main ideas and to understand motives, consequences, cause and effect. This applies particularly to children with specific learning needs, for example those with Autism Spectrum Disorder, Specific Language Impairment and associated learning difficulties.

Reading Between the Lines is designed to help teachers, teaching assistants and speech and language therapists to develop inference skills in their students. It provides a range of graded texts, giving children practice in identifying implied information. It is aimed at children in Key Stage 2 (aged 7–11). It can be used one to one, or in small groups.

How to use this book

Structure of the book

Reading Between the Lines consists of 300 texts which aim to develop inferencing skills in children. At the end of each text the child is asked a key question. The answer can be inferred from the text but is not directly stated. Ten main areas of inference are covered. The five sections in the first half of the book contain texts referring to Action, Place, Occupation, Object and Instrument. The texts in the second half, which deal with Category, Problem–solution, Cause–effect, Time and Character/feelings, are likely to prove more difficult.

The texts in each category are roughly graded in Levels 1–4. Levels 1 and 2 provide many highlighted 'clues', while Levels 3 and 4 contain one or two clues which are not highlighted. There is an introductory activity for each category, which consists of a very brief text.

The levels are not strictly age-related, but follow a broadly developmental sequence, in accordance with Dr Marion Blank's work on children's levels of questioning (Blank *et al*, 1978) . Younger children will not be expected to reach the higher levels. The target for any child is to be able to deal successfully with the texts they are likely to encounter in the classroom.

How to start

Select a category from the first half of the book. Present the introductory picture-supported item to the child, ask the question at the end of the text, and note the result. If the child has no problem with it, move on to the first text at Level 1. After the child has read or listened to the story, ask the key question at the end. If a child is unable to understand the inference at this beginning level, the story can still be used to prompt direct questions whose answer is obvious from the text. This is a first step towards drawing inference. Some older children may be able to go straight away to higher levels, and categories in the second half of the book.

You may want to concentrate on certain categories of inference where the child has had particular difficulty, or to work across several categories concurrently.

Non-readers will need the texts to be read to them, and the majority of younger children will need some help with reading. Older children may have competent reading skills, but still have little ability to draw inference from what they read. They can either read for themselves before being asked the key question, or be asked to read the texts aloud to the adult.

Sometimes there will be more than one possible answer.

Teaching at Levels 1 and 2

Introduce the child to the category theme you have chosen, for instance 'These stories are about WHERE something happens' or 'These are about WHEN something happens.'

The first Level 1 text in every category shows the 'clues' printed in bold, and a series of questions and prompts are suggested. These provide a guide to working with the ensuing texts. If you are reading to children, they can still help to identify the clues in bold by pointing to them, and you can repeat them. Be sure always to ask the final question, 'How do you know?' This not only clarifies where the children's ideas have been confused or inaccurate, but gives them practice in explaining. Children who get the right answer before the end of the texts are probably able to tackle the next level.

Supplementary questions

If a child cannot answer the key question, don't forget that you can ask other questions – refer to the example questions in the first Level 1 texts.

Teaching at Levels 3 and 4

At these levels the 'clues' are not highlighted. You will need to tell the children that they have to read the text or listen to the story, and identify the 'clues' themselves. Ask the target question. If they have read the text themselves, encourage them to use a highlighter to find any 'clues'.

Recording progress

There is an optional record sheet at the end of the book.

The texts are all photocopiable.

Introductory activities

Action

Jamie pedalled really hard, but halfway up the hill he had to get off and push.

What was Jamie doing?

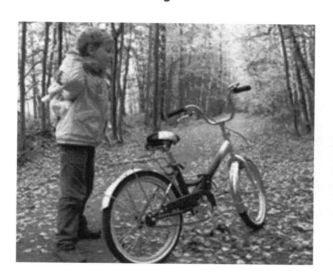
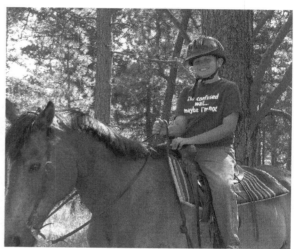

Place

Bobby looked round at the tables, the whiteboard, the computers and the children's pictures on the walls. It was good to be back.

Where was Bobby?

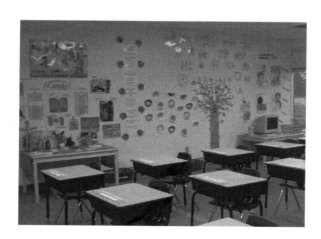
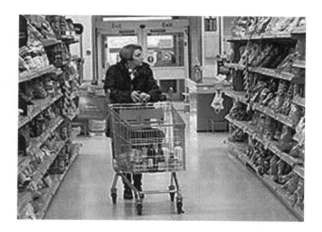

Occupation

Maisy had cut her leg and her mum took her to the hospital accident department. A kind lady in uniform put cream on the cut, and then stuck a plaster on it.

Who was helping Maisy?

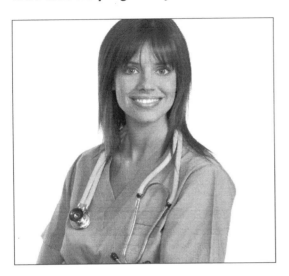 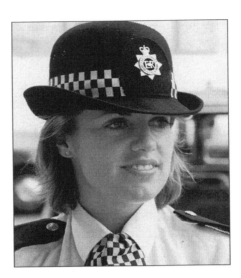

Object

Tommy tipped over the toybox full of cars and bikes and things, and fished out his favourite. It was red and silver, with a big headlight and shiny handlebars.

What was Tommy's favourite toy?

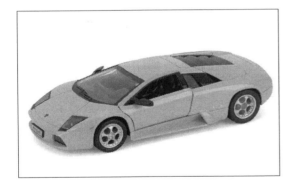 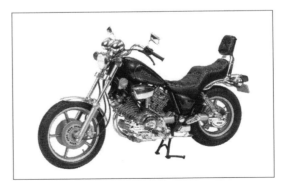

Speechmark

Instrument

Laura's picture was coming on really well, but now she needed to colour some of it in.

What did Laura need next?

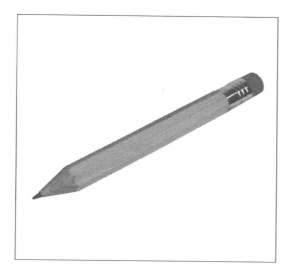

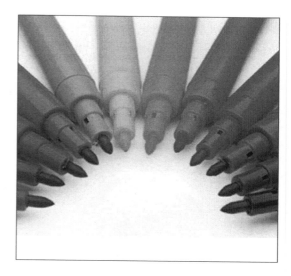

Category

One of the freezers had lots of pies and things in it. The one that Poppy liked was full of Cornettos, lollies, vanilla tubs and Magnums. Just right for a hot day!

What kind of food did Poppy like?

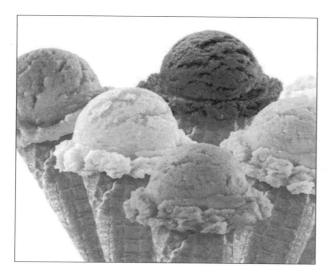

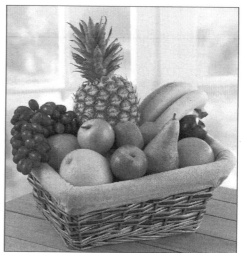

Problem–solution

Mum was on her way to see Gran when the car broke down. Luckily Mum knew just what to do.

What did Mum need to do?

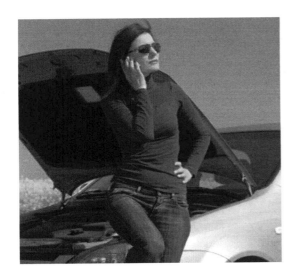

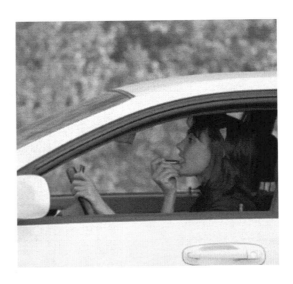

Cause–effect

Emily's new kitten had done something really naughty and Emily was so upset when she saw her fish, and the broken glass on the floor.

What had happened?

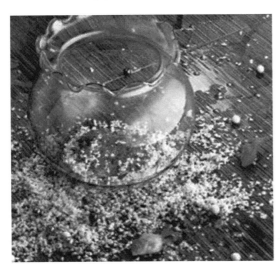

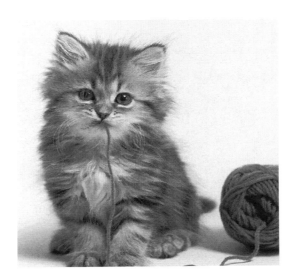

Speechmark

Time

The twins had a lovely bath before Dad came to read them a story in bed.

What time of day was it?

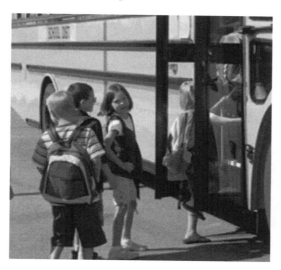 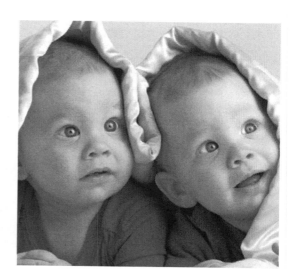

Character/feelings

Rosie didn't like watching her dad doing the garden. She felt so sorry for the worms he dug up, and always tried to rescue them.

What kind of girl was Rosie?

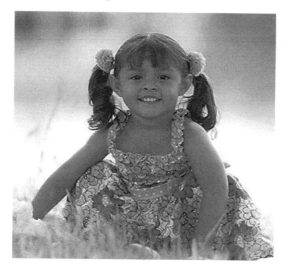 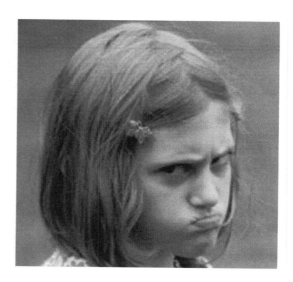

Speechmark

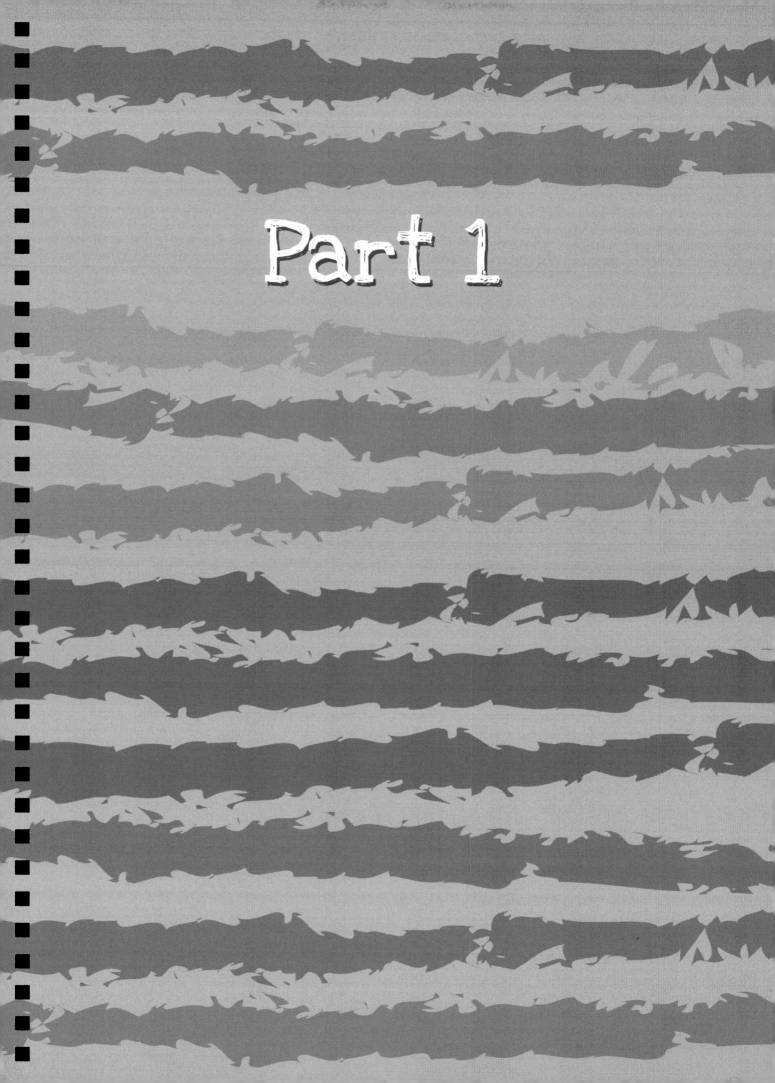

Part 1

Action

Level 1

Find the clues that tell you WHAT'S GOING ON: what people are doing, what's happening.

Clues might be about:

- What people are doing – eating/running/swimming/flying/playing

- What animals or other creatures are doing

- What is going to happen

Here is an example. The clues are in bold type.

Troy and his friends were **playing** out **in the snow**. They **made a snowball**, and rolled it round and round the garden until **it was really huge**. Then they **made a smaller one**, and put it **on top of the big one**. They **stuck two twigs in for arms**, and Troy ran indoors and asked his mum for a **carrot for the nose**. Just then **Troy's dad** strolled out into the garden. He **told them** they **could have his old gardening coat and hat**. The boys ran to fetch the things from the shed. Now all **it needed** was **stones for the eyes and mouth**, and they **stuck some on** carefully. It looked just great. Troy said he'd seen one that had a pipe in its mouth. Nobody knew anyone who smoked a pipe, so they decided they would just have to make a pretend one.

What were Troy and his friends doing? How do you know?

- *The boys were playing in the snow*

- *They made two big snowballs, a big one with a smaller one on top*

- *They stuck twigs in for arms*

- *Ted got a carrot for the nose*

- *They fetched Dad's old coat and hat to dress it in*

- *They stuck stones on for eyes and mouth*

- *They must have been making a snowman*

Story 1

Barry **stood behind Jordan's chair** and **looked** over his head **into the mirror**. 'Hmm,' he said. 'We need to take quite a lot off, I think.' He **fetched a trolley** full of **brushes and combs and scissors**, as well as all sorts of pots and bottles. He **combed** carefully through **Jordan's hair**, to get it into shape, and **reached for the scissors. Soon** there was a **pile of hair on the floor**, and a girl came along to sweep it up. Jordan began to think he soon wouldn't have any left. Then **Barry picked up some clippers**, and **tackled the back of Jordan's neck**. The **clippers buzzed and tickled**. At last Barry said, 'There you are, then.' He **held up a mirror** behind Jordan's head. **Jordan** thought he **looked very trendy**, and much more grown up.

What was Barry doing? How do you know?

Story 2

Daisy opened the cupboard, and **took out flour and sugar**. Then she opened the fridge, and **took out butter and milk**. She **weighed everything**, and **put it into a bowl.** Next she took a wooden spoon, and **began stirring and beating**, until it was all mixed together and lovely and smooth. She ran her finger round the bowl and licked it. Yummy! Then she **squeezed the mixture into a big lump**, plonked it on the work surface and **rolled it flat** with a rolling pin. She **found the cutters**, and **cut out star and moon shapes**. When she had **fitted the shapes on to a baking tray**, she **popped the tray into the oven**. Daisy looked at her watch. She **had to remember to take them out** in about 10 minutes.

What was Daisy doing? How do you know?

Story 3

The group had only been going for about a quarter of an hour, and already they were **beginning to pant and gasp**. 'Phew,' Jason said. 'This is **going to be harder than we thought**.' 'You've done nothing so far,' laughed the leader. 'We've **only come about a quarter of a mile**. **Look back towards the valley** and you'll see.' 'Well, **my legs ache** anyway,' said Mike. '**Some bits are really steep**.' 'Never mind,' said the leader. 'We'll **have a little breather** before we carry on. Look up ahead, and think **what a great view** there will be **when we get to the top**.' The **boys looked up**, and **could see** patches of **snow on** some of **the highest peaks**, up above where the trees stopped. After a few minutes, they struggled to their feet and **plodded on**.

What were the boys doing? How do you know?

Story 4

Jared's new foster mum was great. She had **got Jared a hamster**, which he had always wanted. It was a gorgeous fluffy creature with toffee-brown coloured fur, and Jared had decided to call it Brownie. The deal was that **Jared would do all the work** of looking after him. They had **bought a** lovely **big cage**, and Brownie seemed to have settled in well. Now it was **the first day of Jared's job**. He **collected a brush and a pan**, some **hot soapy water** and a cloth. Then he **opened the cage**, and **popped Brownie into the box** his foster mum had found for him. He **put some food in** there too, so Brownie wouldn't try to escape. Then he **took the dirty water bowl** and **food dish out** of the cage, and **set to work**.

What was Jared going to do? How do you know?

Story 5

It had been raining a lot, and the **sports field was pretty wet**. The **PE teacher** said he **would go** and **have a look**. When **he came back**, he had a **big smile on his face**. 'The **field's not too bad**,' he said. 'We **can go ahead** all right.' The **boys rushed off to change** into their sports gear. They found **Mr Allen laying a tape on the ground** between two pegs. He **told the boys to line up** side by side behind the tape. 'Be careful you **don't put a foot over the tape**, or we'll have to start again,' he said. He **put** his **whistle to his lips**, but before he could blow it **someone had started to run** and had gone over the tape. '**Start again**,' said Mr Allen. '**Ready? Steady?**' And **he blew** a shrill blast **on the whistle**.

What were the boys getting ready to do? How do you know?

Story 6

Ted **looked out of** his bedroom **window**. Something was going on out there. A **red van** with 'FIRE' written on the side **was parked** by the pavement. **Two firemen got out**. They were **carrying a ladder**. Then he **saw Mrs Grimshaw** from Number 19. She was **looking very unhappy**. '**It's Tabitha**,' Mrs Grimshaw was saying. 'She's **always going up trees** and then **she can't get down**.' The firemen looked at each other and grinned. 'Don't cry, Ma,' said one of them. '*We* might get scratched, but *she'll* be all right.' The other **fireman put his foot on** the first rung of **the ladder** and **began to climb**. Ted got dressed as fast as he could, ran downstairs and out of the front door, hoping to get there before all the excitement was over.

What were the men going to do? How do you know?

Level 2

Story 1

Tim threw a pile of clothes on the bed. 'Better start with the most important things first,' he thought, and began **putting in his fleece, ski jacket and ski trousers**. '**Don't forget** the boring things like **underpants and socks and wash things**,' called his mum from downstairs. By the time Tim had put all those in and added his **DS and iPad** to amuse himself **on the flight**, there wasn't much room left and he had to **sit on the lid** to get it shut.

What was Tim doing? How do you know?

Story 2

Looking out of the window, Layla could see Dad **going down the garden with a spade**. He was **carrying something in a carrier bag** in his other hand. Layla **started crying again**, as she thought of her poor little **hamster**. Now she would never see him again. Dad had promised to put up **something to mark his grave**, with his name and the date on it.

What was Layla's dad going to do? How do you know?

Story 3

Johnny put on his **hat with the Jolly Roger** on it. He found the black eye patch, and pulled the elastic band over his head. When it was on, he really **began to look the part**. 'I **just need a parrot** now,' he laughed to himself. 'Just then Mum called up the stairs, 'Hurry up, Johnny. I can hear Pat's dad's car **outside**. **Don't keep them waiting**.'

What was Johnny going to do? How do you know?

Story 4

Grandma **made some sandwiches** and put them in a plastic bag. She **put some buns, biscuits, fruit** and **chocolates in** as well. '**Don't forget the rug**, the **ground may be** a bit **damp**,' said Grandad, as he picked up the **basket of food** and **carried it to the car.**

What were the family going to do? How do you know?

Story 5

A man **wearing a balaclava**, with a **mask over his eyes, walked into the bank**. He **went up to one of the cashiers** behind the grille, and **pulled something out of his pocket**. Some of the **customers screamed**, and **one or two ran out** of the bank into the street. The cashier pressed a secret button under the counter.

What was the man trying to do? How do you know?

Story 6

There had been a terrific gale, and most of **the leaves** on the trees in the garden **had blown down**. The **lawn looked very messy**. After an hour's hard work, Anya **wheeled the last barrowload** up the steps, and **filled the last bin bag**. The **garden looked nice and tidy** now.

What had Anya been doing? How do you know?

Level 3

Story 1

Will crept into the cupboard under the stairs, and pulled the door shut. He could hear the others rushing about the house, looking behind chairs and under the beds. Somebody shouted, 'Cuckoo, we can't find you!' but Will kept quiet.

What were the children doing? How do you know?

Story 2

Noah lay down on the ground and peered into the pond. It was muddy, and he couldn't see anything in there. Still, he pulled his net carefully through the water. When he pulled it up, there were four or five little black wriggly things in it, the size of matchsticks. He tipped them into his jam jar.

What was Noah doing? How do you know?

Story 3

Lydia wriggled until she was inside the sack with her head and arms poking out. The teacher checked to see that the children were in a nice straight line, and blew her whistle. After three steps, Lydia was flat on the ground.

What were Lydia and the other children doing? How do you know?

Story 4

Kasia looked in the mirror to see that her headdress was on straight, and clutched her posy of flowers tightly. The music started to play, and her big sister in her beautiful dress and veil moved towards the church door. Kasia walked solemnly behind her.

What was Kasia going to do? How do you know?

Story 5

The doctor got Adam to sit down on a chair. 'Just a little scratch,' he said to Adam. 'Hold out your arm.' Adam did as he was told, and shut his eyes. He hardly felt it, and the doctor said he had been very brave.

What was the doctor doing? How do you know?

Story 6

Jeff's car started to pull to the left and bump along the road. Jeff knew all the signs. He parked the car on the verge, got the jack out of the boot, and lifted the spare tyre out on to the grass.

What was Jeff going to do? How do you know?

Level 4

Story 1

Mum looked at the pile of muddy rugby clothes lying in a heap on the kitchen floor. Toby had another match tomorrow. Mum picked up the heap with a sigh.

What was Mum going to do? How do you know?

Story 2

Jan finished the plate of sandwiches, and looked around for something else to eat. She was still hungry. She fetched a knife, and opened the forbidden tin .

What was Jan going to do? How do you know?

Story 3

Aaron collected the bundle of newspapers and put them in his bright yellow shoulder bag. He looked at his list of addresses, mounted his bicycle and pedalled away.

What was Aaron going to do? How do you know?

Story 4

Lola opened her eyes and realised that it was morning. She felt disappointed that she wasn't really flying on a magic carpet and wearing those wonderful clothes.

What had Lola been doing? How do you know?

Story 5

Tom washed the mud off the tyres, and looked proudly at his beloved machine. Those scratches really spoilt it. Tom went to fetch the paint.

What was Tom doing? How do you know?

Story 6

'Higher, please!' shouted the little girl, gripping the ropes tightly. Mum gave her a really big push.

What was the little girl doing? How do you know?

Story 7

John pulled the ripcord, the great silk canopy opened up above him, and he began to float gently down.

What was John doing? How do you know?

Story 8

Gary gripped the wheel tightly as they bounced over the waves. Sheets of spray drenched him as he pulled back the throttle.

What was Gary doing? How do you know? Was he going fast?

Story 9

Lisa finished the last one and put away her calculator. She put her name at the bottom of the page. Then she went and waited in line to show it. She did so hope that Miss Robins would be pleased with her again this time.

What had Lisa been doing? How do you know?

Story 10

The leader crawled out from the tunnel into a big space, where stalactites hung dripping down from the ceiling. He shone his powerful torch round in amazement.

What was the leader doing? How do you know? Where was he? What are stalactites?

Story 11

Kane thought about the last time he had been in that room. It was when he had that awful rash, and now his throat was terribly sore. He looked at his watch, and realised it was already nearly 12.

What was Kane doing? How do you know?

Place

Level 1

Find the clues that tell you WHERE IT IS/WHERE IT HAPPENED.

Clues might be about:

- What you can see

- What you can hear or feel

- Places where certain special things happen

Here is an example. The clues are in bold type.

Susie was going on a **trip with her class**, and she was really excited. When they arrived, they went in through a big gate in a high fence. **The first animal** they saw was **an elephant**, eating from a big heap of hay. They could hear some **parrots squawking**, and there was a **cage** where **monkeys** were swinging around on ropes . The monkeys came close to the wire and seemed to want to say hello to the children. Mrs Robinson said it was really important not to feed them. Giving them the wrong food could make them ill. The **seals** had a lovely **big pool to play in**. 'We'll come back here at three o'clock,' Mrs Robinson said. 'Then we can see the **keepers feeding them**, and the **penguins** too.'

Where were they? How do we know?

- *They were on a school trip*

- *They could see and hear wild animals and birds*

- *The animals had special places to live in*

- *There were keepers who fed the seals and the penguins*

- *They must have been at the zoo*

Story 1

At last Billy finished building his **sandcastle**. Mum said, 'Let's go and find some **shells** to put on it.' They walked across the **sand**. Billy liked the smooth wet feel under his bare feet. He found some lovely coloured shells, and decorated his castle with them. Then they dug a ditch all round the castle. Mum said, 'When **the tide comes in**, the ditch will fill up with water and turn the castle into an island. You can stand on the top and be the king of the castle.' Afterwards Billy took his **shrimping net** and fished about in one of the **rock pools**. **He caught** three tiny **crabs**, and put them in his bucket, with plenty of water to keep them cool. Before they went home, Billy put the crabs down on the sand and watched as they raced towards the water. The smallest one got there first.

Where were Billy and his mum? How do you know?

Story 2

Jimmy put his clothes in the **locker**, picked up his **towel** and paddled through the **shower**. When he **got inside**, it was really noisy – there were **shouts, laughter** and **splashing**. He walked carefully so as not to slip on the **wet floors**. He made his way past the water chute to the far end by **the diving board**, where he had to meet the teacher. He was feeling really nervous, and sure he would be the worst in the class. He remembered all the times his dad had tried to get him started, and it had always ended with him spluttering and coughing and his feet still on the bottom. Some quite small **children were swimming** without armbands, and Jimmy made up his mind that this time he was really going to do it.

Where was Jimmy? How do you know?

Story 3

'Come and give me a hand in here,' called Dad, as Freddie ran **down the garden**. 'I've got some jobs to do.' Freddie **went in**. This was his **dad's special place**. He spent hours in there, cleaning and polishing his **spades and forks** until they shone like silver. 'Right,' said Dad, giving Freddie a pile of **small pots**, 'fill these with earth. Press it down firmly. Then put three of these **seeds in each one** and cover them up with more earth.' 'What are they, Dad?' Freddie asked. '**Sunflower seeds**,' said Dad, 'and if you have done your job properly, they **will grow into plants** taller than you. We might even win a prize with one of them.' Freddie set to work, filling each pot and putting the seeds in. When the pots were all filled, he gave the seeds **a gentle watering**. 'You've earned your lunch,' said Dad.

Where were Freddie and his dad? How do you know?

Story 4

Mum **parked the car and collected a trolley**, and they **went inside**. Mum started **putting** all sorts of boring **things** like **washing powder and milk into her trolley**. Molly **wandered off** down one of the aisles and picked up a bar of her favourite chocolate off the shelf. Would Mum let her have it? Then she heard her mum calling, 'Molly! Molly! Where have you got to?' Molly quickly put the chocolate back and started to run towards Mum's voice. Round the **end of an aisle** she **bumped into** a big **stack of baked bean tins**. The tower toppled and the tins rattled to the floor, making the most awful noise. At that moment Mum appeared, flustered and out of breath. 'Oh my goodness, Molly, what on earth have you done?' Molly wished the floor would open up and hide her.

Where were Molly and her mum? How do you know?

Story 5

Josh was bored. He had read all the books Mum and Dad had brought him, and there was nothing worth watching on TV. A **nurse** came in, and Josh called her over. 'Any chance I can **get up** this morning?' he asked. 'Maybe after lunch,' she said. Josh looked at the bed next to him. The bloke in it seemed to spend all his time asleep, so he was no fun. **The bed the other side** had nobody in it: the boy in that one had **gone home** the evening before. Just then a **doctor** came in and strolled down the ward. He stopped by Josh's bed, and Josh braced himself. What was it going to be this time? Another **injection**? 'What do you think of the idea of going home this afternoon?' asked the doctor. 'Really truly?' shouted Josh. 'Really truly,' said the doctor cheerfully, and wandered on down the ward. Josh found he wasn't feeling bored any more.

So where was Josh? How do you know?

Story 6

Mum said, 'We've got half an hour, children. You can all **choose two each**, and meet me back by the **checkout machine**. I'm going to take Rose to the **DVD section**.' The older children set off. Dan was very keen on wildlife, and made his way to the **non-fiction aisles**. Lily went that way too, as she wanted to find out how to grow a sunflower seed for a competition. Ben, the eldest, loved exciting **adventure stories** and went to the **fiction shelves**. When they had all made their choices, they went to the checkout machine, and Ben **showed Dan and Lily how to use it**. Then they went to meet Mum and Rose. Rose was carrying a **DVD of Mary Poppins**. 'She must have seen that DVD about a hundred times,' Dan said, laughing.

So where were the family? How do you know?

Level 2

Story 1

'This is my favourite **shop**,' said Dad, stopping by the window. 'Let's go in and see what they've got today.' Lucy **pushed open the door**. A wonderful **smell of warm bread** greeted her. It was one of her favourite shops too, and she loved Mr Archer who owned it. Mr Archer was always jolly and smiling; he was very fat, and looked as if he ate quite a lot of **his own buns**. Lucy could see some of that day's batch of **buns and cakes** on the counter **behind the glass screen**. They looked simply delicious. Dad didn't usually buy her anything in here because Mum said it would spoil her tea, but Mr Archer sometimes gave her something as a treat. Lucy looked longingly at the buns, and Mr Archer grinned as he popped one in a paper bag. 'Mind you eat your tea, though,' he said, 'or we'll both be in trouble.'

Where were Lucy and her dad? How do you know?

Story 2

They were far too early. Dad would have left it until the last minute, but Mum always liked to have plenty of time. Emma was excited – **two days in London**. There would be so many things to do. She hoped they would fit in a trip on the London Eye, and the pantomime was definitely booked. They waited on the **platform** for what seemed like ages, and Dad checked to make sure they all had their **tickets**. Mum nipped off and bought a magazine to read, and Dad got himself a cup of coffee. 'Do you want anything?' he asked Mum and Emma. They both said no thanks. Emma started to feel rather cold: there was a chilly wind blowing. Just then she heard a sound. 'Hooray,' she said. 'I think I can **hear it coming**!' 'You're right,' said Dad. 'So can I.'

Where were Emma and her parents? How do you know?

Story 3

Mr Armstrong had just written the **number line** on the whiteboard as the bell for **playtime** went. Hakim gave a sigh of relief. He couldn't wait to get outside and spend a bit of time kicking a football around with his friends. He was really hoping to get picked for the first team this year. He knew he was pretty fast. At the last trial he had beaten everybody in the race. Hakim supported Man U, and he had brought in a photo he'd taken when he'd gone with his dad and his brother to see them play. He thought his friends would be really interested when he showed it to them. He stuffed the **numeracy work into his bag**, and joined the rush to the door. Mr Armstrong's voice boomed out behind them, telling them to **walk not run**, and not to make such a noise.

Where was Hakim? How do you know?

Story 4

Sam watched as his uncle tapped the numbers on his ticket into the machine. The light changed from red to green, and Uncle Bob drove slowly forwards between the rails. Then the big machine began to **spray water** all over the **roof** and **sides**. It was noisy and rather frightening, and Sam wished that he could get out. Two huge black and white brushes, looking a bit like pandas, began spinning **against the sides of the car**. Sam shut his eyes, and held Uncle Bob's hand. 'Don't be scared, mate,' Uncle Bob said. 'I've been through here loads of times and I promise you nothing ever goes wrong.' The noise stopped and Sam opened his eyes again. He felt a bit silly when he realised that nothing awful had happened.

Where were Sam and his uncle? How do you know?

Story 5

Adeena and her friends climbed up the great wide staircase to the first floor. At the top they found themselves in a room full of **big glass cases**. The cases held all sorts of **pots** and **vases**; sometimes they were in one piece and sometimes there were **just bits** of them. Adeena didn't find them very interesting, and she wandered off into the next room. This was more like it! The glass cases in here were really huge, and held the skeletons of different **dinosaurs**. She recognised a Tyrannosaurus rex, and a Diplodocus. She was just setting off into the next room to see what was in there, when one of her classmates caught up with her. 'Miss Jackson is wondering where you've got to,' Lucy said. 'You'd better come back right away.'

Where were Adeena and her friends? How do you know?

Story 6

Charlie and Max gazed around. There were so many **rides**, they wondered how they could possibly manage to go on them all. 'Let's go on that **big water slide** first!' Charlie shouted, running towards it. 'There's a **bit of a queue**,' Mum said. 'Should we wait until there aren't so many people?' 'There's a queue because it's the BEST thing,' Charlie said. 'Can we get a packet of crisps and we can eat them while we're waiting?' 'OK,' Mum agreed. 'And we could get Dad to join the queue for the **mystery train** to save us another long wait.' Armed with crisps and bottles of juice, Mum and the boys settled down to wait. From where they stood, they could hear the **excited screams** of people on the water slide, and see the children launching themselves down the **helter-skelter**.

Where were Charlie and Max and the family? How do you know?

Level 3

Story 1

Captain Andrews floated around inside the capsule, checking that everything was in order. As he drifted past the TV, he saw the scientists at the Control Centre staring at their screens. They were watching the tiny dot that was *Mars Explorer*, orbiting the earth.

Where was Captain Andrews? How do you know?

Story 2

Nathan gripped the arms of his seat as the engine roared, and they gathered speed. Then there was a bump, and out of the window he could see, over the wing, the ground getting further and further away.

Where was Nathan? How do you know?

Story 3

Tess remembered the last time she had been in this room. Then it had been Polly who had had a damaged wing. Just then a man in a white coat came into the room. 'Next please,' he said. Tess gripped the basket tightly, and followed the man through the door.

Where was Tess? How do you know?

Story 4

The family found a table by the window and sat down. They passed the menu round. Katie had no trouble making a decision. She chose her favourite, fish and chips, and sticky toffee pudding for dessert.

Where were the family? How do you know?

Story 5

The lights went down until it was nearly dark. Everything was quiet except for the rustling of popcorn bags and one or two people coughing. Then a shimmering castle appeared on the screen, and soft music began to play.

Where was this? How do you know?

Story 6

Hassan held his sister's hand as they climbed the stairs and made their way right to the front. There were two empty seats. It was fun being able to see into the upstairs windows of shops and houses. Hassan pretended to be the driver.

Where were Hassan and his sister? How do you know?

Level 4

Story 1

Mr and Mrs Ashworth collected the key from the reception desk, and went up to the second floor in the lift. Their room was lovely, with a view right over the harbour.

Where were they? How do you know?

Story 2

A brilliant kick sent the ball flying into the goal, passing the goalie's outstretched hands by inches. The home supporters let out a mighty cheer, and waved their banners.

Where were they? How do you know?

Story 3

The family waited in line to have their passports checked. Gemma was so excited to think that in just two hours they would be in Spain.

Where were they? How do you know?

Story 4

The man had walked for hours. At last he sat down on the sand, and watched as the tide came in.

Where was he? How do you know?

Story 5

It was so lovely to be there. They lay in bed watching the regular flash of the lighthouse through the window.

Where were they? How do you know?

Story 6

Daisy was unpacking her suitcase. There was still sand in her shoes, and she lifted out the little bag of shells. She wished she were back there on holiday.

Where had she been on holiday? How do you know?

Story 7

The audience held their breath as the man stepped on to the wire high above their heads, and began to inch along it. 'Thank goodness there's a net to catch him if he falls,' said Grandma.

Where were they? How do you know?

Story 8

Maddy went gingerly down the steps at the shallow end, launched herself on to the rubber ring, and swallowed a mouthful of water.

Where was she? How do you know?

Story 9

'Don't be such a baby, Susie,' Mum said. 'The man's only going to look at your teeth this time.'

Where were they? How do you know?

Story 10

'They're the only ones I like, and Mum says the heels are too high,' Betsy said crossly.

Where were they? How do you know?

Story 11

George looked down the row of beds just like the one he was in, and realised he hadn't dreamt the accident after all.

Where was George? How do you know?

Story 12

Jenny smashed the ball over the net, and ran up to shake her opponent's hand as a storm of clapping broke out.

Where were they? How do you know?

Occupation

Level 1

Find the clues that tell you WHAT SOMEONE'S JOB OR HOBBY IS.

Clues might be about:

- Where they work

- What they like doing

- What sort of work they are doing

- What they are making

Here is an example. The clues are given in bold type.

Rory was feeling happy. It was Friday, and on Friday nights he and the others always met at Joey's house. Joey was allowed to **practise in the garage**, which was huge. There were electric sockets to **plug the gear into**, and enough room for Joey's **drum kit**. His parents didn't mind how much **noise** they made. After school, Rory set off, the heavy case **slung over his shoulder**. This week he had learnt some new **chords**, and was looking forward to showing the others. When he got to Joey's, the others were already there and everyone was very excited. 'Guess what?' said Joey. 'We've been asked to do a **gig at the school disco**!'

What was the boys' hobby? How do you know?

- *The boys needed somewhere to practise*

- *They needed to plug things into the electric sockets*

- *There was a drum kit*

- *Rory had something in a case*

- *He'd learnt new chords*

- *They had been asked to play at a gig*

- *The boys were in a band*

Story 1

It was still pitch **dark** when Matt heard the alarm go off. He yawned, sat up and looked at the clock. **Half past five**. Better get a move on: he had a lot on today. He quickly put on his **overalls**, splashed some cold water on his face and went down to the kitchen. He made a thick cheese and pickle sandwich and a flask of tea. Bess was in her basket, **wagging her tail**. Then he put on his **wellies** and a dark green jacket, picked up his lunch box and he and Bess set off . As he walked down to the yard, it was just beginning to get light. When he reached the **milking parlour**, he switched on the lights and checked the machines. Then he walked up the lane to the **field** at the top of the hill, Bess running ahead. As he reached the gate, he whistled at her and she immediately stopped and lay down beside the gate. He could just see the **herd**, gathered at the fence, waiting. As he opened the gate, he could feel the **warm breath** of the ones in front.

What was Matt's job? How do you know?

Story 2

It was Tom's favourite place. He loved the peaceful **river**, the willows on the far bank, and the sound of the weir further downstream. The little **boat** was tied in its usual place. Tom climbed in, bailed out the water in the bottom and mopped the seats dry. Then he opened the wicker basket and laid out **all his gear** on the middle seat. He had learnt how to choose the best places from his dad. His dad was an expert, and had been a good teacher. When he was ready, Tom lifted the **rod** and flicked the fly out **over the water**. It was already beginning to get dark when he reached home that evening. 'Any luck?' called his dad from the living room. '**Three**!' Tom called back triumphantly. '**Enough for dinner!**' It had been a really great day.

What was Tom's hobby? How do you know?

Story 3

It was a cold, windy afternoon. Mum and Robbie walked over to Granny's house for tea. They knocked on the door, and soon Granny appeared. She kissed Robbie on the top of his head and said, 'Perfect timing – we can check I've **made the sleeves** the right length.' He followed her into the sitting room. The fire was lit and it was lovely and warm. Granny opened her bag with the pink and red flowers on it and pulled out several funny-shaped pieces, which she **held up against** him. First his **back**, then his **front**, then each arm. One of the pieces was still attached to the **needle** and Granny said, 'Right, I need to do about **four more rows** on this one.' She put the other pieces back into the bag, picked up another needle and carried on, her **fingers moving so fast** Robbie could hardly see them. And all the time she was chattering away to Mum without even looking at what she was doing. Robbie wondered how on earth she could do that.

What was Granny's hobby? How do you know?

Story 4

Mum took the iPad into the kitchen and propped it against the bread bin. Then she got a stool and climbed up to reach the top shelf of the cupboard. She took out the things she needed, one by one, and put them on the worktop. Then she got down off the chair and slid it back under the table. The next job was to **switch on the oven**. Gas Mark 6 it said in **the recipe**. There was a sound of footsteps coming down the stairs. 'Me do helping,' said a little voice. Tom was nearly three and he loved mixing things and stirring in the kitchen. 'Come on, then,' said Mum, reaching for a big bowl and a wooden spoon. She carefully **measured flour**, sugar and butter and put them in the bowl. Then she broke three eggs and added them to the mixture. She gave Tom the wooden spoon and let him have a stir. When it was all mixed up, she poured it into two round tins and **put them in the oven**.

What was Mum doing? How do you know?

Story 5

Miss Sharp went into the charity shop. They had lots, stored on the shelf at the back. She didn't like the really big ones, because they took so long. Five hundred was about the **right number of pieces**. She looked along the shelves. At the end there were three that were just right. Now she had to **choose which picture**. The ones with pretty cottages were always nice to do. Or maybe a seaside village. In the end she decided to get one with a view of a windmill in Holland. It was raining hard when she got outside, so she caught the bus home. She cleared off the end of the big table in the dining room and **opened the box**. Then she **tipped the pieces** on to a tray and turned them all the right way up. 'Corners and **straight edges first**,' she said to herself as she started to sort out the pieces. 'There's an awful lot of sky in this one,' she thought.

What was Miss Sharp's hobby? How do you know?

Story 6

Laura opened her eyes. The room was brighter than usual. She looked at the clock. 'Oh no!' she thought as she leapt out of bed. 'The alarm didn't go off! It's half past already and I'm going to be **so late**.' She washed and dressed as quickly as possible. There was no time for breakfast, so she shoved a banana in her bag, grabbed the car keys and slammed the door behind her. As she drove through the busy morning traffic, she suddenly remembered that she was supposed to be **taking Assembly** today. Not only that, but there was a **new boy** starting who had arrived from Germany only last week and apparently didn't speak any English. She was thinking about **who she could ask to be his buddy** and make him feel at home, when she also remembered it was her turn on **playground duty**. Laura finally drove through the gates into the car park thinking, 'What a **bad start to the week**.'

What was Laura's job? How do you know?

Level 2

Story 1

Mr Mack walked through the door. In the background he could hear **barking** and a cat **miaowing**. 'Any problems with any of them?' he said. Emma looked up from the screen. 'Scamp keeps trying to **lick his scar** and poor old Mog won't eat anything at all this morning,' she replied. Mr Mack put on his **white coat**. He washed his hands and looked at the list on his computer screen. 'Help,' he thought. 'How am I going to get to see all of them and get out to Apple Tree Farm to **check that bull** before 12 o'clock?' Just then there was a tap on the door. Emma said, 'Mrs Bunting is here with Flossie.' 'Right, send her in then,' said Mr Mack. Mrs Bunting came in carrying a wicker basket. An angry **growling noise** came from inside the basket. 'Put the basket on the table, Mrs Bunting, and let's take a look at Flossie.' Mrs Bunting opened the door of the basket. There was a hiss, and a large grey **cat jumped** straight off the table and went and hid under the trolley.

What was Mr Mack's job? How do you know?

Story 2

Tom wheeled his bike out of the shed. It was a cold, wet morning. He **slung the empty bag** over his shoulder and rode down the road to the row of shops. 'Hi there, Tom,' said Mr Naseem. 'You're late again; that's the second time this week.' 'Sorry, Mr Naseem,' he replied. 'I won't be late again, I promise.' He went round the back of the counter to the little storeroom. Ben was already there, **filling up his bag**. He passed Tom a huge **bundle**. Tom stuffed them in the bag and he and Ben walked out of the shop together. '**Which road are you doing?**' said Ben. 'Porter Street,' said Tom, frowning. 'It's uphill all the way so there's no point taking my bike.' He set off on foot. Some houses had a special **box for papers** by their gate. Others, he had to **push it through the letterbox** or leave it in the front porch.

What was Tom's job? How do you know?

Speechmark

Story 3

The afternoon went really slowly. The last lesson was Maths and Miss Riley's voice seemed to go on for ever. Magda couldn't see the point of 'estimating' how many marbles there were in a bag. She could perfectly well count them, and then it would be right. As soon as the bell went, she hurried down to the cloakroom and **changed into her kit**. She walked across the school **playing field**, right to the top where the **courts** were. None of the others were there yet. Magda was feeling a bit nervous because today Mr Lee was going to pick the players for the **tournament**. Magda took her **racquet** out of her bag and **practised a few strokes** while she was waiting.

What was Magda's hobby? How do you know?

Story 4

Sue Brown opened the door and rushed in, saying sorry for being late. 'That's OK,' said Kali, taking her coat and holding out a black gown to put on. They walked through into the **salon**, and Kali showed Sue where to sit. 'So, what are we doing today, Mrs Brown?' asked Kali. Sue looked at herself **in the mirror** and frowned. 'I'm not sure. What do you think?' she said. 'Maybe make it **shorter at the sides** and **tidy up the back**,' said Kali. Sue agreed and Kali asked her to walk over to the basins. She sat down, **leaned her head back** and relaxed. When Kali had finished and had wrapped the towel round, Sue followed her back to the chair. She sat down and picked up a magazine while Kali **picked up the scissors** and got to work.

What was Kali's job? How do you know?

Story 5

It was a wet day. Outside in the street people were hurrying along with umbrellas up. The windows were beginning to steam up. Jen checked to make sure all the **tables were laid**. The door opened and a woman came in, pushing a buggy. Behind her were two small girls. They must be twins, thought Jen, because they looked exactly the same. A crying sound came from the buggy. The woman looked tired and fed up, and the little girls were beginning to push each other. 'Hey, let me help,' said Jen. She beckoned to the little girls and **led them to a table** at the back. 'Right, you two, sit here and have a look at the **menu**. What would you like?' The mother lifted the crying baby out of the buggy and he stopped straight away. She joined the girls at the table and looked at Jen. 'It's been one of those days,' she said. 'I'd like **a big cup of coffee**, please, and the girls would like **juice and a cake** each.'

What was Jen's job? How do you know?

Story 6

Jim's phone alarm woke him. He got out of bed and quickly put on his **uniform**, grabbed his keys and ran down the stairs. Outside it was dark and very cold. The windows of the car were covered in ice and he had to scrape it off before he could see to drive. He set off, driving as fast as he dared on the icy road. Soon he arrived at the station. Several other cars were just pulling into the car park. They all rushed into the station and **grabbed their helmets**. 'It's at Number 24 Chestnut Drive,' said the boss. 'Get there as quick as you can: we don't want it to spread **to the house next door**.' Jim was the driver. He climbed quickly into the cab and reversed out of the station. Once they were on the road, he turned the **siren** on. There was one set of traffic lights and they were red, but this was an emergency. Jim drove straight through as fast as he could.

What was Jim's job? How do you know?

Level 3

Story 1

He stepped back and wiped the brush on an old rag. It needed more blue, so he reached for the tube and squeezed out a small blob. 'Too bright,' he muttered, and added a tiny bit of grey. Then he took a smaller brush and carefully dipped it in the blue-grey mix.

What was his hobby? How do you know?

Story 2

'That should be enough,' she said, cutting through the slices so that there were two piles of triangles. She wrapped them in silver foil and put them in a plastic bag. 'They can go in the fridge till the morning.' Then she cleared up the crusts and bits of cheese and lettuce, and put them in the bin. She stacked the pile of sandwiches on the counter.

What was her job? How do you know?

Story 3

Mark looked at his list of jobs for Tuesday. First he had to cut Mrs Owen's grass. Then he was helping Mr Biggs at Number 17 dig a new pond. After that, he had three different people's hedges to clip. If he got through all that, he might have time to go and plant the big flowerbed at Lime Tree Cottage. He went to his shed and collected all his tools.

What was Mark's job? How do you know?

Story 4

First she folded it in half. Then she took one of the pieces of coloured card and drew the shape of a teddy. She cut it out and stuck it on to the front half. There were some coloured stars in the packet, so she stuck them along the top. Underneath the teddy she drew some flowers. Then she opened it up and got her gel pens to do the writing on the inside.

What was her hobby? How do you know?

Story 5

Alan knocked on the door of Number 10. 'Morning, Mrs Cotton. I'm ready to start. I'll just go back to the van to get my stuff.' In a few minutes he was inside Mrs Cotton's new kitchen. He put his equipment down on the floor. 'Now, are you sure about the colour?' he asked, looking at the paint chart in Mrs Cotton's hand. 'Yes,' said Mrs Cotton. 'That duck egg blue is exactly right.' Alan got the brushes ready and opened the first tin. Then he went back to the van for the stepladder for the tops of the walls.

What was Alan's job? How do you know?

Story 6

Kyle was shopping with Aunt Floss. He hoped Floss might buy him the new one to add to his collection. Kyle was very proud of his collection. He had 59 now, all piled carefully in his room in the right order. None missing since he had started collecting. His favourite character was always on the front page, and he loved the pages where readers sent in their own pictures. And, of course, the stickers to add to his sticker album. This week there was a free toy stuck to the front. It looked like some kind of boat.

What did Kyle collect? How do you know?

Level 4

Story 1

She wrote the date on the board and turned to face the class. 'Today we are going to see what happened to the cress seeds we planted last week,' she said.

What was her job? How do you know?

Story 2

Mum put the heavy plastic basket down on the grass. One by one she lifted the wet sheets out and hung them up. 'Good thing there's a breeze,' she said. 'Should be dry in no time.'

What was Mum doing? How do you know?

Story 3

He cut two slices and put them on the plate. He couldn't decide whether to have cheese and pickle or ham ones today, but when he looked in the fridge, there wasn't any ham left. 'Have to be cheese and pickle, then,' he said, picking up the knife.

What was he doing? How do you know?

Story 4

Mr Trim raised the chair to the right height by pressing a lever with his foot. Then he tilted the mirror to the right angle. 'OK, Mrs Mills,' he said. 'Open wide and let's have a look at what's causing all this trouble.'

What was Mr Trim's job? How do you know?

Story 5

'Three burgers, a Coke and two coffees, please,' said the man at the table. Rich quickly wrote it on his pad and went to the next table.

What was Rich's job? How do you know?

Story 6

Hattie opened the oven door. 'Mmmm, that smells good,' she said, lifting the tins out. When they had cooled down a bit, she carefully turned them out on to a wire rack. 'Now for the icing,' she said.

What was Hattie making? How do you know?

Story 7

Jamil opened the basket and lifted him out. 'He won't eat anything and he just lies there. He doesn't even want to chase the cat,' he said unhappily. 'What do you think's wrong?'

Who was Jamil talking to? How do you know?

Story 8

'What about down there, in that shady bit by the river?' They all agreed that was the best spot, so they walked down the hill, carrying the basket and the coolbox. When they got there, they spread the rug on the ground and opened the basket.

What were they doing? How do you know?

Story 9

Malik parked on the clifftop, got changed, picked up his board and headed for the shoreline. Perfect weather for it, a bit of a wind and some big waves developing.

What was Malik's hobby? How do you know?

Story 10

Ginny had one last look in her dressing room mirror. She put just a touch more lipstick on and straightened her wig. She always felt nervous just before she went on, but no need, really. She knew her lines, and the last rehearsal had gone well.

What was Ginny doing? How do you know?

Story 11

Ed spoke softly to the horse as they circled the paddock for the last time. 'This is the big one, old fellow,' he whispered. 'Go like the wind!' They followed the rest of the field to the starting line.

What was Ed's job? How do you know?

Story 12

Meg put on the bright yellow jacket, picked up the 'Stop!' sign and walked up to the school gates just as the children started to come out. When there was a gap in the traffic, she stepped out, holding up the sign, and let the first ones cross.

What was Meg's job? How do you know?

Object

Level 1

Find the clues that tell you WHAT IT IS.

'What is it?' clues might be about:

- What the thing looks like – big/little, shiny, pointy

- What the thing feels/sounds/smells like

- What the thing is used for/what it can do/what different parts it has/what it's made of

It might be a person, a creature or a thing.

Here is an example. The clues are in bold type.

Sal stared round the **shop**. They all looked so wonderful, with their **shiny metal wheels** and the coloured **stripes on the frames**. It was really hard to choose. 'The size is important,' Dave said. 'Not too small, or you'll grow out of it in no time. Not too big, or you won't be able to reach the **pedals**!' The assistant brought out one that looked just right. Sal tried sitting on it while Dave held it steady. He showed her how the **gears** worked, and which levers to squeeze to put the **brakes** on. 'You'll need a **bell**,' the salesman said, 'so everyone will hear you coming!' They also bought a **light** for the **front handlebars**. Sal **pushed it** home proudly. The whole family came out to watch her when she had her **first ride** on it in the park.

What did Sal get? How do you know?

- *Sal was in a shop*

- *She was looking at things with shiny metal wheels and stripes on their frames*

- *They had pedals, gears and brakes*

- *Sal bought a bell, and a light for the handlebars*

- *Sal pushed the thing home and then she had a ride on it*

- *It must have been a bike*

Story 1

'This is the one you are going to **ride** today,' said Mandy, the teacher, leading him out. 'His name is Bilbo.' Tilly stroked his **soft nose**. 'Can I give him a bit of **carrot**?' she asked, 'I've got some in my pocket.' 'Of course you can,' said Mandy. 'He'll be your friend for ever.' Tilly held her hand out flat with the carrot on it, and Bilbo gently picked it off with his lips. His **whiskers** tickled Tilly's hand. 'He's lovely,' said Tilly. 'Shall I get his **saddle**?' 'Yes please,' said Mandy. Tilly fetched the saddle, put it on Bilbo and fastened the **girth** tightly round his fat tummy. Mandy put on the **bridle** and gave Tilly a leg up. Tilly put her feet in the **stirrups**, gave Bilbo a gentle **kick**, and he set off obediently towards the **paddock**. Tilly felt excited. Maybe today she would learn to **canter**!

What was Bilbo? How do you know?

Story 2

Ben was in the **pet shop** to choose his birthday present. He was looking at a **big empty glass box**, but Ben knew when he had finished his shopping it would hold a magical world. The shop assistant showed him one that was already **filled with water**, with **bubbles rising up** from the air machine. 'The fish like to be able **to hide** sometimes,' the shop assistant said, 'so you might like to **have a tunnel for them**.' Ben got one, and some of the right **water plants**. Now to **get his first fish**! He chose **brilliant blue neons** and **two guppies**. Ben was about to pay for it all when the shopman stopped him. 'Haven't you forgotten something? They won't last long if you don't feed them!' Ben was so embarrassed! He bought plenty of fish food, and carried everything out to Dad's car.

What was Ben buying? How do you know?

Story 3

A crowd was standing on the pavement, looking up at the **church tower** and the big, round **face** on its side. The **numbers round** the edge of the face were in black curly writing, and the **hands** looked as if they were made of gold. 'It's over three hundred years old,' the guide said. 'And it still **keeps perfect time**. It will **strike in a minute**.' The face opened, and two little figures came out with a gong and hammers. They raised their hammers, there was a wheezing noise and a click, and the **dwarves struck the gong three times**. Tess **looked at her watch – exactly three o'clock. 'Does it do the half hours** too?' she asked. 'No, **only the hours**,' the guide said. 'So if you want to watch it again, come back just before four.' 'Just time for something to drink and a sticky bun first, then,' said Mum.

What was Tess looking at? How do you know?

Story 4

The picnic was finished, and the grown-ups were packing it away. 'Buzz off and amuse yourselves for a bit,' Dad said. 'We're going to have a little snooze in the sun.' The children ran off. Harry called out, 'Come over here! This would be **a great one for climbing**!' They all looked up where Harry was pointing. As they looked, **a squirrel scampered up it**. The **branches were big**, but some of the **lower ones were smaller** and **easy to reach**. '**You're the best climber**, Harry,' everyone agreed. 'You have a go and see if you can do it.' **Harry jumped** and **caught hold of the lowest branch**. With a heave he **pulled himself up** until he was sitting on it. A **shower of leaves** fell down on the children as the branch shook, and they laughed. 'Go on, Harry! See **how far up you can go**!' they said.

What was Harry climbing on? How do you know?

Story 5

The boys settled down in the back row to **wait for the film to begin**. It was the new James Bond, and they were all excited. 'I reckon we **should eat them right away**,' said Will. '**Who's got them**?' '**Me**,' said Nick. '**Shall I pop the bag**?' 'Yes, go on,' said Gary, 'might as well **make the noise now** before the film starts.' **Nick clapped his hands together** and the **bag burst** with a **loud pop**. He passed it along to the others, and they **all took a handful** and **started chewing**. It **sounded awfully loud**, and a **lady in the next row** turned round and **glared at them, saying 'Sh!'** in a fierce whisper. 'Eat them quickly,' whispered Gary, 'or she'll get us thrown out.' The boys tried not to giggle as they finished them up.

What were the boys eating? How do you know?

Story 6

The Robinson family had **moved to a new house**. It was completely empty, no furniture and no curtains or carpets. While they were waiting for the van to arrive with their own stuff, the children **set off to explore**. They tried all the doors downstairs and found nothing but spiders. Then they moved on to the upstairs rooms. In the very last room they found a small door in a corner. They all had a go at tugging on the handle, but it was really stiff. They twisted and turned it, and pulled some more. They were just about to give up when Freddie gave a last heave, **the door flew open**, and Freddie fell over backwards. An avalanche of things came tumbling out – **teddy bears**, **Dinky cars**, **bits of LEGO®** and mysterious boxes that rattled. 'Wow,' said Freddie. 'Treasure trove!'

What did the children find? How do you know?

Level 2

Story 1

Annie's **uncle** was a **pilot**. He flew businessmen to meetings all over the UK and over to France, Holland, Belgium and Germany. Today Annie's dad had brought her to meet Uncle Ted as he landed back from a trip. They **waited on the tarmac**. 'There he comes,' said Dad suddenly, and pointed. Uncle Ted **landed** neatly only about **50 metres away**. The **draught from the rotor blades** blew Annie's hair about, and the noise was deafening.

What landed on the tarmac? How do you know?

Story 2

'Hey, come and **look at this one**,' said Tommy, giggling. He showed it to his sister. 'I **took it off Grandpa** when he wasn't looking. He **was fast asleep in his chair**, and his mouth was wide open, and he was snoring really loudly.' Meg came over to see, and she began to laugh too. 'You'd better not show Grandpa,' she said. 'He might be really upset. He always pretends he doesn't fall asleep after lunch.' Tommy **pressed the forward button**.

What did Tommy show Meg? How do you know?

Story 3

Lucy took the box. 'Can you guess what it is?' asked Aunt Bessie. The box was square, and not very heavy. It could have been all sorts of things. 'Give me a clue,' she said. 'Right,' said Aunt Bessie, 'you were talking about needing a new one just a few days ago. This is a very new model. I've paid for a **month of calls** for you, and **it's a camera as well**.' 'I know what it is!' shouted Lucy excitedly, and began ripping off the pretty paper to get at the box. 'Wait till I show my friends at school. I'll **text my best friend** right away.'

What was Lucy's present? How do you know?

Story 4

Dave **put** the **last two pieces in** with a shout of triumph. The **picture** of a harbour full of boats was **complete**. The box and **all the pieces** had **been lying on the table** in the hall since before Christmas, and **everyone** had been **putting a piece or two** in when they went past. Dave was really chuffed to be the one to finish it. It was the hardest one he had ever done, with **a thousand pieces**, and lots of sky and clouds, so **loads of the pieces** looked **nearly the same**.

What was Dave making? How do you know?

Story 5

Arvan was helping his mum to **put the shopping away** in the kitchen. It was a very boring job, but at the same time you needed to concentrate. You had to sort out what should go in the fridge, what in the cupboard under the sink and what in the store cupboard. At last he got to the **bottom of the big shopping bag**, and **fished out** the **last box**. It felt **very cold**. 'Oh, **good**,' he said. '**Vanilla. My favourite**.' Well, don't stand there looking at it,' said his mum. 'Put it **in the freezer before it melts**.'

What had Arvan taken out of the shopping bag? How do you know?

Story 6

Nan was slicing carrots. Suddenly she gave a little shriek, and held up a finger dripping with blood. 'Oh, how careless of me,' she said. 'I was doing all the things I tell you children not to do when you are cutting anything.' Nan wound a bit of kitchen paper tightly round her finger, and she and Tilly went upstairs to the bathroom. 'You'll have to strap it for me,' she said. 'I can't manage with one hand.' Tilly got the little **box** out of the **bathroom cabinet** and **cut off a strip**. She wound it carefully round Nan's finger and **pressed it to make it stick**. 'How does that feel?' she asked.

What did Tilly put on Nan's finger? How do you know?

Level 3

Story 1

Maya peeped into the bottom of the cupboard. Muffet was in the basket, purring loudly, and cuddled up beside her were four tiny bundles of black and white fluff. Maya gently picked one up and held it carefully. It just fitted into her hand.

What did Maya see in the cupboard? How do you know?

Story 2

Dad had been building something in his shed. He said it was a surprise. When they looked out of the window in the morning, they saw what the surprise was. Mum had hung some nuts on it, and put out seeds and some bits of bread. Two bluetits and a robin had already arrived for breakfast.

What had Dad been building? How do you know?

Story 3

Grandpa was prowling about the house, turning over books and papers, looking in drawer, and muttering. 'I've lost them again. Oh bother; I'm always losing them,' he was saying to himself. Karen started laughing. 'Grandpa, they've been on your nose all the time,' she said.

What had Grandpa lost? How do you know?

Story 4

Halfway up the M4 the driver started to look worried. 'I've forgotten which is the best turn-off,' he said. 'There's one route that is much better than the other. Can you pass me that big yellow book from the back seat, so I can look it up?'

What sort of book did the driver want? How do you know?

Story 5

Dad was on the phone. He kept saying, 'Yes, yes ... OK, yes. I understand. Hang on a minute ... ' He beckoned to Dean, who was listening. 'I need something to write this down with, Dean,' he said. 'Thanks. OK, carry on,' he said into the phone.

What did Dad want Dean to give him? How do you know?

Story 6

The family piled out of the car and unloaded all the luggage. They carted it up to the front door. It had been a long drive, and they were all tired, hungry and thirsty. Dad was standing by the door patting his pockets. 'Where on earth are they?' he said. 'At this rate we'll have to get back in the car and spend the night in a hotel.'

What had Dad lost? How do you know?

Level 4

Story 1

The dog was barking at the bottom of the hedge, where a small bright-eyed creature was rolling itself up into a ball.

What was the dog barking at? How do you know?

Story 2

As the dark clouds rolled in and the first drops began to fall, Marylin felt in her shopping bag and pulled out the bright red new one she had just bought.

What did Marylin take out of her shopping bag? How do you know?

Story 3

The beautiful creature slowly spread out its gorgeous fan-like tail, shimmering blue and bronze and green, and stalked away.

What was the creature? How do you know?

Story 4

There on the table sat the chef's masterpiece, covered with white icing, and five candles burning brightly on top.

What was on the table? How do you know?

Story 5

Nathan put it to his eyes, adjusted the right eyepiece, and suddenly the distant view came into sharp focus.

What was Nathan looking through? How do you know?

Story 6

Gran opened the heavy volume and began to turn the pages, exclaiming in delight as she followed the life of her grandchild from babyhood to the present day.

What was Gran looking at? How do you know?

Story 7

In the distance the hero saw the grey shape of a man gliding across the grass. It seemed to be wearing a cloak and hood, and Jem found he could see right through it.

What did the hero see in the distance? How do you know?

Story 8

Jon gazed up at the sky. He could not see anything, but he could just hear the faint noise of the engine, and see a growing line of white smoke against the blue.

What could Jon see in the sky? How do you know?

Story 9

'Goodness,' said Lily as Gran put the snowdrops in it. 'I must have made that when I was about ten!'

What was Lily looking at? How do you know?

Story 10

As it gathered speed, trees, houses, lakes and tiny stations flew past in a flash and the children stared out of the window in excitement.

What were the children in? How do you know?

Story 11

Dad switched the car engine off. Lots of cars had stopped in front of them. In the distance they could see the top of a huge lorry, and there was a blue flashing light.

What might there be ahead of them? What makes you think so?

Story 12

Samantha would always remember how she felt at the end, when she sat on the throne, with the crown on her head and the beautiful robe, and the audience clapped and clapped.

What was Samantha remembering? How do you know?

Instrument

Level 1

Find the clues that tell you WHAT SOMEONE WAS USING or WHAT THEY NEEDED.

Clues might be about:

- Things people need

- Things people use at home or at work

Here is an example. The clues are in bold type.

Dad was very pleased with his birthday present. 'That's a really good one,' he said, taking hold of the two **handles** and **wheeling** it round the garage. He bent down to look at the front **wheel**. 'Good strong **tyre**, that is,' he said. 'Come on, Micky. You can have a **ride** up to the allotment in it; then you can help me **load it** with vegetables.' He lifted Micky in, took hold of the **handles** and they set off up the road. Later that morning, Mum saw them on their way back. Dad looked hot as he **pushed** it through the gate. It was piled high with potatoes, courgettes and carrots.

What was Dad using? How do you know?

- *It had two handles*

- *It had wheels*

- *It had something to do with gardening*

- *It was big enough for a small boy to ride in*

- *You can put lots of things in it and push it along*

- *It must have been a wheelbarrow*

Story 1

It was Billy's birthday. He was six. His mum said, 'Come and look outside, Billy. See what's in the garden.' She opened the back door and Billy looked. There it was, on the path. 'Wow,' said Billy. 'Wow, it's a proper big boy's one! Can I have a go right now?' Mum said he had to get dressed and put shoes on. So he ran up the stairs and put on his top and shorts and a pair of wellies that didn't really fit any more. Then he went into the garden to have a good look. The **handlebars** and **seat** were green and the **wheels** were really shiny. On the back, behind the big wheel, were two small wheels. 'That will help you **balance**,' said his mum.

What did Billy have for his birthday? How do you know?

Story 2

'At last,' said Maisie, smiling. She had just finished writing a story about the Celts. She had to pretend she was a Celtic girl and write about her day. She had found some really good pictures on the internet and her brother had shown her how to copy and paste them into her story. It was looking good and she was pleased with her work. She reached in the cupboard for some more **paper** and slid it into place. Then she pushed the lead into the little slot in the side of the **laptop**. As soon as she did this an **orange light** began to flash. 'Oh no,' said Maisie. '**It's run out of ink!**' She called upstairs to her brother. 'Tom, have we got another **cartridge**? Will you **load it** for me, please?'

What was Maisie having trouble with? How do you know?

Story 3

RikEE2 touched the screen and a large Chocolate Shooting Star with Orbit Sprinkles appeared. 'Yummy,' he said as his mouth filled with the delicious creamy ice cream full of crunchy sprinkles. When he had finished the last mouthful, he turned around and walked towards a big crater. There were lots of little craters and he had to look carefully to make sure he didn't get his foot stuck in one**. 'I just hope it will start this time**,' he said to himself. '**It didn't sound quite right when we landed**.' RikEE2 was looking forward to getting back to Kraz and seeing his family. At last he reached the big crater. There it was, waiting round the back. It was silver with a **round glass dome.** As RikEE2 came nearer, a **green light started to flash** and the **shiny doors slid open** silently.

What had RikEE2 left behind in the crater? How do you know?

Story 4

It was Friday afternoon. Laura was sitting at her table trying really hard to listen to Mr Budd talking about how tadpoles turn into frogs. It was a hot day and she wanted to be outside. 'Right,' said Mr Budd, 'open your books and draw the life cycle of a frog, starting with the frogspawn. Then colour it in carefully.' Laura was pleased to have a chance to use her new felt pens. She reached across the table and picked something up. It was a new one, with Barbie on the outside. She **unzipped** it. Inside there were **pencils**, **felt pens**, a **rubber** and a **sharpener**. They all fitted into their own little space in neat lines. She took out a pencil and the rubber and all the felt pens. Then she **zipped** it up again.

What did Laura pick up? How do you know?

Story 5

Dad loved making things. Last week Mum had been moaning because there were too many books in the sitting room. 'There isn't enough room on the shelves,' she said. 'Don't worry,' said Dad. 'I'll put up some new ones.' So this morning he went off in the car and came back a bit later with the boot open. Three long bits of wood were poking out of the back. 'This won't take long,' he said cheerfully. He went into the shed and came back with his hands full. I helped him carry the bits of wood into the house. 'The first job is to **make the holes in the wall**,' he said. He got a pencil and marked where the shelves would go. Then he **plugged** it in and fixed a short **pointed metal thing into the front**. He was just about to press the **start button** when Mum said, 'Stop! You haven't checked where the electricity wires go!'

What was Dad using? How do you know?

Story 6

Jake looked out of the window. A big lorry had stopped by the front gate. Two men got out and opened the back. They lifted a huge cardboard box out and put it on the pavement. Then one of the men came and knocked on the door. Mum opened the door. 'Great!' she said. 'Bring it into the kitchen.' They slit open the sides of the box with a knife and took away the cardboard. It was tall, much taller than the old one. Mum opened the door. 'Oooh, look!' she said. 'It's got a box at the bottom to keep the **vegetables** in and a special **drinks dispenser**. And that dial tells you when the **temperature** is too warm. You don't have to **defrost** this one either: it does it on its own.'

What did the lorry deliver? How do you know?

Level 2

Story 1

Milo was a wizard. He lived in a funny little house at the end of the street. The door was painted with blue and red stripes. Milo was really good at reading stories to children. He was so good at it that Hilltop Primary School asked him to do their Story Club every Friday morning. Every Friday he chose a book and walked up the hill to the school. He sat on the floor with his legs crossed, just like the children. Sometimes he sang a song with strange words that no one could say. Sometimes he took something out of his bag, **waved it around** and said, '**Abracadabra!**' When everyone was looking at him, he started to read. One Friday Milo woke up late. He had to rush off to school without having his breakfast. He was in such a hurry that he forgot to take a book. 'Never mind,' he said to himself, reaching into his bag. But, oh dear, all he found was an old apple core, three rubber bands and a spare wizard's hat. Wherever could it be? He had last used it **when the fire wouldn't light** two days before.

What did Milo use every day? How do you know?

Story 2

Milly was excited. In five days it would be her seventh birthday. But something weird was going on. Every night, after tea, Dad went off to the shed. She could hear him **sawing and banging** and sometimes she heard the sound of a drill. 'He's definitely **making something**,' she thought. One evening she heard Mum and Dad talking after she had gone to bed. 'I know,' said Mum, 'I could use **wrapping paper**...' Milly couldn't hear the rest of the sentence. She got out of bed and tiptoed over to the door and listened again. 'No, that would be too thick,' said Dad's voice. '**Maybe Nan could knit one**. Anyway, I've only got a couple more bits to do. It will definitely be finished in time.' At last it was Saturday, Milly's birthday. She went into Mum and Dad's room. In the corner was a very big present. Milly tore off the paper and gasped. 'Wow, it's amazing,' she said, bending down to peer inside. 'Oh look, a **rug** and **wallpaper** and real **curtains**!'

What did Mum and Dad make for Milly's birthday? How do you know?

Story 3

Josh and Tom walked down the little path to the beach. The tide was a long way out, but you could still see the big waves crashing on to the shore and the tiny dots that were people surfing. On the wide, flat beach there were people walking their dogs. Big white clouds **raced** across the sky, and every now and then someone's hat would **blow away**. 'Brilliant day for it,' said Tom as they carefully unzipped the bag and laid it out on the sand. 'You go first,' said Josh and he carried it away, towards the shoreline. Tom made sure there was nothing twisted, and then waved his arms and shouted, 'Ready!' Josh picked it up and ran towards Tom before **launching it upwards**.

What did Josh and Tom take to the beach? How do you know?

Story 4

When Petra woke up, there was an odd white light in the room. She pulled back the curtains and gasped. The whole street was white. Big, silent snowflakes were falling and settling on the road, the cars, the rooftops, the trees. Everything was white. Downstairs Petra's mum was listening to the local radio. After a bit she looked up, smiling. 'Guess what, Pet?' she said. 'School's closed because of the snow – you've got the day off!' Petra skipped around the kitchen in excitement, then ran upstairs and dressed in her warmest clothes. Then she went into the garage. **It was stored on a shelf**, too high for her to reach. 'Mum,' she called, 'I can't reach it. Can you come and get it down?' Mum got a stepladder and climbed high enough to grab the front. She pulled it down, dusted it off and said, 'Right, let's get out there, shall we?' They trudged **up the hill**, Mum in front, pulling it behind her. Finally they got to the top. Petra turned it round, sat down and **held on to the wooden sides**. Mum gave her a push and she was **zooming** through the snow.

What did Petra take up the hill? How do you know?

Story 5

Grandad said if you stood at the highest point of the hill and looked towards the river, you might see a kingfisher. Ellie had seen kingfishers in a book. Beautiful little birds with bright blue feathers. The book said they were shy birds and you didn't see them very often. Ellie really really wanted to see one. Grandad liked going for walks and was keen on birdwatching, so on Saturday they set off up the hill. 'Here you are. **Put the strap round your neck** and don't let them bang into anything.' Ellie walked carefully, one hand holding the strap to keep it steady. When they got to the top, Grandad put his hand on Ellie's arm and pointed. '**Hold them up to your eyes** now, keep still and look carefully.' Ellie did as she was told. After a little while, she saw a flash of blue through the **lens**.

What did Ellie use to see the bird? How do you know?

Story 6

Billy and Jo were staying with Nana. She lived in a big house in the country. The first day it was pouring with rain, so they couldn't go outside and play on the swing or climb trees in the orchard. Nana said, 'Never mind, boys. I know what you can do. You can go up to the attic. There are lots of interesting things up there. Take this: you might need it. I'm not sure **if the lights work up there**.' Billy and Jo climbed up the ladder and pushed open the door. Jo grabbed Billy's arm. 'It's too dark, I'm scared,' he said. 'Oh come on, Jo. Don't be a baby, it's fine.' They took a few careful steps into the dark space. Then Billy tripped over something. 'Ouch,' he said as he got up. '**I'd better turn this on**.' Nothing happened. '**Maybe it needs new batteries**,' said Jo.

What needed new batteries? How do you know?

Level 3

Story 1

Connor lined up with the other children, holding it tightly in his hand. It was a birthday present from his Auntie Pat. Auntie Pat knew he loved Fireman Sam, so she chose a really good present. 'Right, Year 1, come and sit down.' Connor followed the others and sat at the long table. He undid the zip and took out the sandwich and the crisps.

What did Auntie Pat give Connor for his birthday? How do you know?

Story 2

Fin heard his mum talking to Nan. 'Look, I'll tell Fin to come over and help you. He's brilliant at that kind of thing.' So that afternoon Fin opened Nan's back door and walked in. She was sitting at the kitchen table looking a bit puzzled. 'Oh Fin, I'm so glad you've come to help me. I'm hopeless at this kind of thing. Your mum said this one would be simple for me to use, but I can't even work out how to turn it on!' Fin took it from her and pushed a little button on the side. The screen lit up. 'Right, Nan,' he said, 'see the little green button on this side. That's the one you press to answer it.'

What was Nan having trouble with? How do you know?

Story 3

Jan had a brilliant idea for her little boy's fourth birthday cake. She decided to make a robot, because little Ned loved them. She made a list of all the things she needed for the cake. Then she drew a sketch of what she wanted it to look like. It needed a square for the head and a rectangle for the body. She opened the cupboard. There were loads of different sizes, but they were all round. So she phoned the special cake-making shop in town. 'I need a square one and a rectangular one, please,' she said.

What did Jan need for the cake? How do you know?

Story 4

Billy was very excited. This was going to be the best birthday treat ever. They were going by train, because Mum had said the skate park was only a short walk from the station. Billy's best friends, Alfie and Sanjay, were going to meet them at the station. At last it was time to go. Billy tucked his skateboard under one arm and carefully held the little black case in his other hand. 'I think it would be better if I carried it in my bag, just till we get there,' said Mum. Billy's eyes lit up. 'If it's good enough, I could put it on YouTube,' he said.

What did Billy take to the skate park? How do you know?

Story 5

It was a really hot day, so Mum told Ellie and Gemma they could have the paddling pool out. They took turns to pump up the four rings until you could see the dolphin pattern on the sides. Mum said, 'Right, ready to fill up now!' 'Me first!' begged Gemma. 'OK, calm down. You can both have a turn,' said Mum. 'And don't forget to rinse off all the dust and cobwebs first.' Gemma grabbed the end but, before she aimed it at the pool, she pretended it was a karaoke machine and started to sing into it. Ellie was too busy turning on the tap by the wall to notice, and suddenly there was a shout as water spurted straight into Gemma's face.

What was Gemma using when her face got wet? How do you know?

Story 6

Carlo sat on the chair in the optician's office. The optician turned out the lights, except for one bright one shining on the letters on the wall. He told Carlo to read as many letters as he could, starting with the big ones at the top. Next the optician put a metal thing with holes on to Carlo's nose. He put different bits of glass into the empty holes and asked Carlo which one made the letters clearer. It seemed to take ages, and Carlo was getting a bit bored. Finally the optician said to Mum, 'You and Carlo choose a frame; then we can order them and you can collect them next week.'

What did Carlo need? How do you know?

Level 4

Story 1

Uncle Jim was putting up shelves in his garden shed. Billy was helping him. 'Billy, can you pass it up so I can put these screws in?' he said, holding a long screw between his teeth.

What tool did Uncle Jim need? How do you know?

Story 2

Mum looked at the pile of shirts in the washing basket. 'Phew, it's going to take ages to get through that lot,' she said to herself. She plugged it in and turned it up to *hot* and started on the pile.

What did Mum plug in? How do you know?

Story 3

'Right, Year 4, you need to listen carefully. Today you are going to measure the height of all the cupboards in the classroom and find out which is the tallest. Come and take one of these each and let's get started.'

What are the children using? How do you know?

Story 4

Anna curled up on the sofa and sniffed. Her mum put her hand on Anna's forehead. 'It feels a bit hot; I think you might have a temperature. Let's take it and see. Open your mouth.'

What did Mum put in Anna's mouth? How do you know?

Story 5

Jeff went into the greenhouse to check his lettuce plants. The leaves were drooping and the soil felt dry. 'Just in time,' he said to himself, filling it from the water butt.

What was Jeff using? How do you know?

Story 6

The girls were busy making Easter cards. They had drawn eggs and chicks and lots of flowers on the front. 'Let's use the ones in the tin,' said May. 'The colours are much better.'

What were the girls using? How do you know?

Story 7

'I think there's a piece missing,' announced Laura. 'There can't be,' said her cousin, Katie. 'We only just opened the box. It must be there somewhere. Have another look. It's going to have some blue and a bit of green for that tree.'

What did Laura think was missing? How do you know?

Story 8

The boys had cleared a big space in the middle of the room. They had tipped all the bits out of the box and now they were busy with the layout, trying to use all the pieces. Beside them the engines were waiting to be put in position.

What were the boys playing with? How do you know?

Story 9

'It's no good: I can't open it,' said Dad. He had tried all the ones on the ring but they didn't fit. 'Hey, what about this set?' said Erin. 'That one on the end looks like it might fit.' Dad put it in and turned. Magic! At last they could get in!

What was Dad using? How do you know?

Story 10

Maya finished making her cheese sandwich. Then she got a bag of crisps and a banana and put the whole lot inside. This one had a rather tricky clip to make it shut, but at least nothing could leak out.

Where did Maya put her sandwich? How do you know?

Story 11

Anya really wanted to get the 'Swim Like a Fish' badge, but to do that you had to go underwater. So, here she was, all ready in her swimsuit. All she had to do now was put them on. She stretched the elastic bit over her head and took a deep breath.

What was Anya using? How do you know?

Story 12

Dad lit the campfire and found a pan, a tin of beans and some bread. The boys were starving after the long walk up to the campsite. Jez couldn't wait for a plate of beans on toast. 'Uh-oh,' said Dad. 'That's the one thing I forgot. How are we going to get the tin open now?'

What did Dad forget? How do you know?

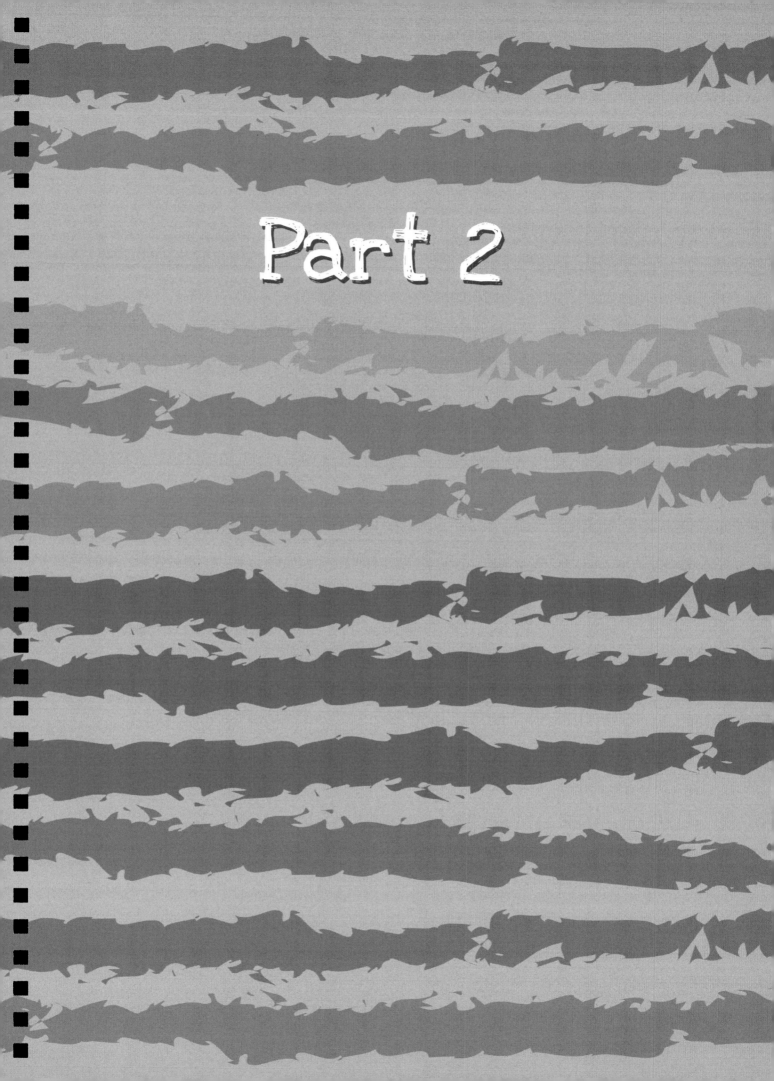

Part 2

Category

Level 1

Find the clues that tell you WHAT CATEGORY (what kind of thing) it is, e.g. animals, furniture, vehicles.

Clues might be about:

• What it looks like

• What you do with it

• Where you find it

• What it's for

Here is an example. The clues are in bold type.

On Saturdays Amber sometimes went to help her Auntie Pat at the shop. She loved arranging everything in the glass cabinet so that the customers could choose their favourites. Auntie Pat usually let her choose where to put the different kinds. Today she decided to start with the **currant ones**, in a row. Then she made a row of the round ones with **pink icing**. She put the lemon ones in the fancy paper cases on a pretty plate on top of the counter. 'Keep the **doughnuts** separate,' called Auntie Pat from the kitchen. 'I don't want sugar everywhere.'

Where did Amber help Auntie Pat? How do you know?

• *Auntie Pat had a shop*

• *There were lots of different kinds, some with currants, some with icing*

• *There were doughnuts*

• *It must have been a cake shop*

Story 1

Maggie was busy in her bedroom sorting toys out. She had spread them out all over the bedroom floor. Now she was putting them into different groups. All the proper baby **ones with soft bodies** were put on the bed. She lined up the **ones with long hair** on the rug. Then she found all the ones with opening and shutting **eyes** and sat them by her cupboard. Next she put the four **boy ones** in a box by the door. She wasn't sure if she wanted to keep them. Maybe her brother Ricky would like them. Finally she put the **ones that came from different countries** on the shelf above the fireplace.

What was Maggie sorting out? How do you know?

Story 2

Mrs Pippin took a big glass bowl out of the cupboard. She fetched her sharpest knife and tipped everything out of the bag into the sink. Then she ran the tap and rinsed everything. After that she took the whole lot over to her chopping board. 'Right,' she said to herself, 'I'll need about four of those, **cut up into little pieces**. And I suppose they will need to be **peeled** first. That lot will need the **pips taken out too**.' She picked up the knife and **starting peeling and chopping**. When she had done all of them, she tipped them into the bowl. Then she went to the fridge and took out some plastic boxes from the supermarket. She carefully pulled back the plastic film from each box and tipped the contents into the big bowl. 'Those look really **juicy**,' she said, popping one that fell on to the table into her mouth. The bowl was nearly full now. Mrs Pippin took a can down from the cupboard, opened it and poured that into the bowl too. 'I'd better taste it to **see if it needs more sugar**,' she said.

What was Mrs Pippin cutting up? How do you know?

Story 3

'Have you got these in black, please?' asked Carly. 'I'll go and check,' said the woman in the shop. She disappeared through a door. Carly carried on looking round the shop. She picked up some really lovely brown ones, but shook her head when she saw the price. Far too expensive. After a while the woman came back with two **boxes**. '**Take a seat**,' she said to Carly. Carly sat down and **tried one on**. It looked good, so she put the **other one on**. Then she got up and walked down to the end of the shop where there was a mirror. 'They look great,' she said as she walked back to her seat. 'The trouble is, they **don't feel comfortable**. Do you have a bigger size?' The woman shook her head. 'I'm afraid not in the black. But I've got them in dark grey or brown.' '**OK, I'll try them on**,' answered Carly.

What was Carly trying on? How do you know?

Story 4

Jenny had a big pile of ironing to do: dresses, sheets, trousers. She switched on the radio and made a cup of tea before she started. Then she put the ironing board up and put the iron on. 'I don't know why Chris has to have a **clean one every single day**,' she grumbled. 'Some days he has more than one. I bet he wouldn't if he was the one that did the ironing.' She sighed and picked up the first one. **Long sleeves** with a stiff **collar** and blue and white **stripes**. It was the one he wore when he went to meetings. The next one had short **sleeves**. It was light blue and he wore it under his patterned jumper when he played golf. Then there were four white ones, the plain sort that he wore to work. Last there was the holiday one. It had a bright pattern of palm trees and boats all over it. Just then the door opened and Chris walked in. 'I've got a meeting tonight,' he said. 'Is it ready for me **to wear**?' Jenny handed it to him, saying, 'From now on I'm going to buy **non-iron** ones.'

What was Jenny ironing? How do you know?

Story 5

Dad answered the phone. Josh could hear him saying, 'Do you think you could deliver it to my address, please?' Then Josh heard him telling the person where they lived. 'Is it coming today, Dad?' asked Josh in an excited voice. 'Yes, they are bringing it over later on this morning. If everything's OK, we can **go round** to show Nana later.' The morning seemed to go very slowly. Josh played on the Wii for a bit. Then he went on his Xbox, but he couldn't really concentrate. At last there was a knock at the door. Josh followed Dad into the hall. The man standing at the door asked Dad to sign a bit of paper. Then he said, 'Right, let's go and check it's all OK.' The three of them went down the front path and opened the gate on to the pavement. 'Wow, **I love the colour**,' said Josh. '**How fast does it go?**' Dad was busy looking through the windows. He asked the man if he could look under the **bonnet**. Then he **got in** and adjusted the seat.

What was delivered to Josh's house? How do you know?

Story 6

Leela and Jamilla were very excited. Today was the day they were going to get their very first pet! They drove up a long drive. At the end was a big house and next to the house were some long, low buildings and a small shed. Outside the shed there was a sign that read 'OFFICE. PLEASE RING AND WAIT'. Mum rang the bell and soon a lady appeared. She was carrying a bucket in one hand and several **leads** in the other. 'Come into the office, then I'll show you around,' she said, smiling at the two girls. When she and Mum had finished the boring paper stuff, the woman said, 'Right, girls, let's go and see what we've got!' They followed her into the first of the low buildings. Inside it was divided up into little pens. They stopped at the first one. 'Ahhh, Mum, he's so sweet!' said Leela. 'Look, he likes me,' she said as the **animal** came over and **tried to lick Leela's hand** through the bars. 'Mum, Mum, I want this one,' called Jamilla, pointing to a black and white one with **big sad eyes and floppy ears**. 'Just remember: you will have to **take him for a walk** every single day,' said Mum.

What kind of pet were the girls choosing? How do you know?

Level 2

Story 1

Shelley was on holiday with her mum and dad. They were staying in a caravan in a place called the New Forest. On the first day they walked along the path that led through the trees. Soon they came to another open space with short grass and some spiky bushes. 'Look over there, Shelley,' said her dad, pointing towards the bushes. That was when Shelley first saw them. **Some brown, some black**. Shelley could see lots of animals grazing, standing in the sunshine and twitching when flies landed on their noses. There was a baby one with **long, wobbly legs** and a white spot on its face. Shelley wanted to go and touch it but Dad said no, because it would be scared. Just then a car went past on the main road and they stopped **munching grass**, looked up and **trotted off** into the distance.

What did Shelley and her dad see? How do you know?

Story 2

Ben seemed to have been standing in the queue for ages. The sun was really hot now, and he couldn't wait to go and sit in the shade for a bit. 'Ben looked at the brightly coloured pictures on the side of the ice cream van. It was really hard to choose, there were so many different kinds. The girl in front of him had chosen a red, yellow and green stripy one in the shape of a **rocket**. Ben's little sister, Amy, wanted **chocolate**, of course. At last it was Ben's turn. 'Yes, young man?' said the lady, smiling down at him. 'Which one do you want?' Ben pointed to the one at the top, in the middle. He couldn't read the writing. 'Right,' said the lady, 'one **Starburst Twizzle** for you, then!' Mum handed her the money and they walked over to a bench in the shade. Amy's was already **dripping** on to her lap.

What did Ben and Amy buy? How do you know?

Story 3

Billy was proud of his collection of vehicles. He had nearly a hundred now. He kept them in a box under his bed. At the weekends he got them out and arranged them on his bedroom floor. There were lots of different kinds. Some had **doors that opened**. He liked those best because you could see inside, and the best ones had all the proper things in them, just like real ones, only really tiny. Billy's little brother, Dan, always wanted to come and join in, but he was annoying because he just wanted to take them away, and then they'd get lost. So Billy shut the door and put a chair in front of it, so Dan couldn't get in. Today he decided to put all the **sporty ones** together, then the old bashed-up ones that used to be Dad's. The rest he lined up in rows, according to **what make** they were. Then he looked at them and wondered what sort he would have when he was old enough to **drive**.

What was Billy playing with? How do you know?

Story 4

Laura was feeling nervous. She had never gone in for a competition before. Her nan had persuaded her to do it. 'Go on, Laura. You are brilliant at it: you'll make a lovely one!' So Laura's mum helped her fill in the entry form for the Portwick Village Show. Today was the day of the show and Laura was busy in the kitchen. Her entry for the competition **was in the oven**. When it had cooled down enough, she had to **decorate** it. She'd decided to make it like a beach scene, with sea, sand, a surfboard and a sandcastle. It took ages to make all the little bits, but finally it was ready. She lifted it on to a special board and her mum carried it to the car. 'Don't worry,' said Mum. 'I'll drive slowly so we don't bump it around too much!' When they got there, Mum carried it to the tent and put it by their number. There were lots of other entries, all beautifully **decorated**, with all kinds of different **icing**.

What was Laura making for the competition? How do you know?

Story 5

The shop had been there for as long as Sharif could remember. He loved looking in the windows on his way to school, and he longed for the day when he could buy one of his own. That wouldn't be for ages though, not until he had a job. His mum sometimes paid him to do jobs in the house for her, but that was only enough for comics and sweets. He stood for a bit, looking in the window. There were some different ones today, but the one he really liked was still there at the side of the window. It was a **racing** one. Everything about it was sleek and narrow, designed for **speed**. Sharif imagined being in the team, covering **mile after mile**, the **wind in his face**, his feet **moving like lightning**.

What did the shop sell? How do you know?

Story 6

Ash and his friend Kyle walked down the steep path. Ash carried a plastic bucket with a couple of bags inside. Kyle had the **tools** and something to eat and drink in a bag. 'My cousin said that's the best place,' said Ash, pointing to a gap in the rocks at the base of the cliff. They finally reached the spot and put the bags and bucket down on a flat bit of rock. 'Let's just have a look around first,' said Kyle. For the next few minutes the boys walked slowly between the rocks, **peering closely** at the ground. Occasionally one of them would bend down and run his hands over the **surface of the rock**. After a bit Ash called out, 'Hey, Kyle, come and look over here!' The two boys crouched down to examine a pile of rocks that had fallen from the cliff. 'Wow,' said Kyle, 'there are at least **three different kinds**!' Ash came back with the bag of **tools** and they set to work **chipping** them out of the rock.

What were the boys looking for? How do you know?

Level 3

Story 1

Ally went into Nanny's garden and sat on the bench with her favourite book, *Fairies and Unicorns*. She'd got to the bit where they were going to have a party. There was a lovely picture of them all in floaty dresses, flying about with their sparkly wings. Ally began to feel sleepy and her eyes began to droop; then something made her open them. She looked up in astonishment. It had sparkly wings, a floaty dress and long, fair hair.

What did Ally see in the garden? How do you know?

Story 2

Miss Plum was planning her Science lesson for Year 3. She had been to the supermarket and bought as many different kinds as she could find. 'That's it; we'll use all our senses to find out as much information as we can. On Friday we'll put the whole lot in a big bowl,' she said to herself. Then she typed a note to herself, *'New words – peel, slice, pips, stones, sweet, sour.'*

What were the children going to try? How do you know?

Story 3

Rob and Nikki followed Dan Brent inside. This one had high ceilings and a view across the valley. Nikki liked the big, light rooms and the amazing bathroom. Rob was excited because there was room for a workshop outside. Nikki began to feel quite excited. At last they might have found the right one!

What were Rob and Nikki looking at? How do you know?

Story 4

Mel walked up to the lady at the counter. 'Please can I look at those over there?' There were so many different styles, it was really hard to choose. Then she saw them. They were silver with three little coloured stones set into them. 'Can I look at that pair?' she asked. She held one up to her ear and the stones twinkled. 'Perfect,' thought Mel. 'They will go with everything.'

What was Mel buying? How do you know?

Story 5

Fin and Lisa loved their pets. Fin had a white rat called Flook and two hamsters called Bubble and Squeak. Their cage needed cleaning out every week. Lisa didn't have to clean out where her pets lived. They didn't smell, they didn't make a noise and they were beautiful to watch as they glided around through the weeds and past the pretend shipwreck.

What pets did Lisa have? How do you know?

Story 6

Jez had to do his Geography homework. He had a fact sheet to fill in. It shouldn't take too long before he could get back to his PlayStation game, which he thought was much more important. He pulled the crumpled-up sheet out of his backpack and smoothed it out on the table while the laptop started up. There was a list of things he had to find out:

Which is the longest in the world?

Which is the widest in the world?

Which is the longest in North America?

How long is it?

What are they important for?

What are the dangers if people throw their rubbish into them?

How can we stop them getting polluted?

What was Jez's homework all about? How do you know?

Level 4

Story 1

Abby ordered them. She asked for three jam ones, two with raisins and four with cream inside.

What was Abby ordering? How do you know?

Story 2

There were two under the log and another four or five scuttling about in the leaves. 'It's easy to scuttle when you've got six legs,' muttered Liam, looking through his magnifying glass.

What did Liam find? How do you know?

Story 3

'So, do you want self-catering, bed and breakfast or full board?' asked the man on the phone. 'Remember, it's cheaper if you get a family room. And where do you want to go from?'

What were they booking? How do you know?

Story 4

Basically there were two types – plant eaters and meat eaters. Some of them lived in damp, swampy places and hunted for food by day and night. They lived on Earth over 200 million years ago.

What were they? How do you know?

Story 5

Jamie didn't know which sort to choose. There were so many in the shop. Big ones, small ones, some with hard covers, some with no pictures. Funny ones, scary ones and chapter ones.

What was Jamie choosing? How do you know?

Story 6

'I need eight animals, one for each child. Then there must be an adult to lead them and another adult to walk alongside. Make sure you choose the quiet ones, I don't want anyone bolting.'

What is the person choosing? How do you know?

Story 7

Kaya peered through the wire fence. There were three baby ones playing in the sun. They looked so cute. She thought the next cage was empty, but then she saw it right at the back, eating a banana. And there was something else, scuttling about in the leaves.

What kind of thing was Kaya looking at? How do you know?

Story 8

The boys stood by the harbour, counting how many different kinds they could see. Some had tall masts; some were tiny with nowhere to sleep. The best were the huge ones you could cross the Atlantic in.

What were the boys looking at? How do you know?

Story 9

Mr Trim loved his garden. So did his neighbours, especially when he left a basket on the doorstep with a sign reading 'Help yourself – take some to go with your Sunday roast!'

What did Mr Trim leave out for the neighbours? How do you know?

Story 10

She emptied her card and photo drawer on the table and started to sort them into groups – ones of the family, ones of holidays, ones of when the children were babies. When they were sorted, she took the new album off the shelf.

What was she sorting out? How do you know?

Story 11

'Why do you need so many different kinds?' asked Nina's younger brother, looking at all the bottles in the bathroom cupboard. Nina sighed: boys just didn't get it. 'Because when you wash it this one makes it shiny, that one makes it smooth and those give a hint of colour.'

What did Nina have so many kinds of? How do you know?

Story 12

Lyla flicked through the TV and radio guide to see what was on. Soaps, documentaries, reality programmes, films, sitcoms and current affairs. She had to write about one for homework. It was hard to choose.

What kind of thing did Lyla have to write about for homework? How do you know?

Problem – Solution

Level 1

Find the clues that tell you WHAT THE PROBLEM IS and think about HOW TO SOLVE IT.

Clues might be about:

- What people are doing – eating/running/swimming/flying/playing

- What animals or other creatures are doing

- What is going to happen

Here is an example. The clues are in bold type.

Rafi was very excited. His uncle Mustafa had given him a brilliant kite for his birthday. It was in the shape of a dragon with a long, fluttering tail of red, green and blue triangles. Rafi couldn't wait to have a go with it. On Saturday morning he took it to the park next to his house. It was a windy day, just right for flying a kite. Rafi's friend Billy came with him. Billy took the kite to the other side of the park and stopped by the big oak tree. Rafi let the string out and Billy threw the kite upwards. It lifted on a gust of wind and soared upwards. But the **wind stopped suddenly** and the kite drifted down, down and down until **it met the top branches of the oak tree**. The string wound itself round some of the small branches and the **kite rested against the leaves**. Rafi stood, holding the string, looking upwards. He didn't know what to do. Just then the man who mowed the grass in the park came by and **stopped his mower right under the tree**.

What was Rafi's problem?

- *His kite was stuck in a tree*

- *It was too high up to reach*

- *The wind had stopped blowing*

- *So his brand new kite was stuck up a tree and he couldn't get it down*

- *What could he do about it?*

- *The man with the mower had just parked it under the tree – maybe it was high enough for Rafi to reach the kite*

Story 1

Mrs Jones put the heavy shopping bag down on the step. She was tired from the long walk up the hill from town and **she couldn't wait to get inside** and make a cup of tea. The sky was getting darker and she felt the first few spots of rain. She dug around in her handbag, but couldn't find what she was looking for. There were lots of other things – her purse, half a packet of mints, sunglasses, her mobile, broken reading glasses and the garage door key. It was raining quite hard now and she was getting cross and wet. Just then Tibs, her cat, jumped through the catflap. He hated being out in the rain. Mrs Jones looked through the window to see where he had gone. She hoped he wouldn't go upstairs with muddy paws. It was then that **she noticed it** lying on the window sill inside. **How on earth was she going to get in now?**

What was Mrs Jones's problem? How do you know? What was the solution?

Story 2

Ben was a bit fed up when his best friend Jan told him he was going to stay with his grandparents in Poland for most of the summer holidays. They were up in Jan's room, playing with Jan's train set. It was a brilliant set with a really big track that was quite hard to fit together. Jan's mum told Jan he had to pack it away while they went on holiday. 'Tell you what,' said Jan. 'Why don't you borrow it while I'm away? You can take it home today.' Ben was pleased. They packed up the track and put it in the box. **'Careful: the box is a bit broken,'** warned Jan. Ben set off up the road to his house. It was a big box, quite awkward to carry. He pushed open the door and put the box on the table. Then he **noticed that one of the flaps at the end of the box was open**. He went up to his room and started to put the track together. After a while, he **discovered he couldn't fit the whole track together**. There seemed to **be bits missing**. Ben couldn't understand it. It had been fine at Jan's house.

What was Ben's problem? How do you know? How did he sort it out?

Story 3

Once upon a time there was a huge hippo who lived by a deep blue lake in the middle of the jungle. He loved spending the long, hot days in the water where it was cool. But he was a mean hippo. He didn't let the other animals come and swim or drink the water. They had to walk a long way to a muddy little pond just to get a drink. One morning they heard a howling noise. It was the hippo. He was lying under a tree **holding the side of his face**, moaning loudly. Just then a little water rat appeared. He went right up to the hippo and said, '**Open wide!**' The other animals watched. They thought the rat was very brave. He crawled into the hippo's huge **mouth**. A few minutes later they heard him say, 'Got it!' and he jumped on to the ground, holding something in both paws. 'You should **feel much better now**,' he said. After that, the hippo made friends with all the animals, but his best friend was always the water rat.

What was the hippo's problem? How did it get sorted out? How do you know?

Story 4

Tyler looked up into the branches of the tree. It was no good: he just wasn't tall enough to reach the lowest branch. If only he could get hold of that branch, he could swing himself up into the tree. **The noise was getting louder now**. 'It's OK. Don't worry, I'm coming,' called Tyler up into the green. '**Just hang on there!**' He didn't know what to do. Mum and Mark were at work and his brother wasn't home from school yet. He walked round to the other side of the house. There was a man in the garden next door standing on **a stepladder**. Tyler went over to the fence and said, 'Excuse me. Do you think you could help me **get up that tree** in our garden?' The man smiled, stepped on to the ground and picked up the stepladder. He carried it round into Tyler's garden and propped it against the tree. 'It's **still up there**, all right,' he said as Tyler disappeared into the branches. A few minutes later he climbed down, **carefully holding the little thing** in his hands.

What was Tyler's problem? How do you know?

Story 5

'Oh no! There's only one here. Mia, have you been borrowing my stuff again? Oh what am I going to do? He'll be here in a minute and I've got to **wear them**!' Laura was Mia's sister. She was 16 and her boyfriend was called Mac. 'Where did you last have them?' she asked her sister. 'They were in my room, I'm sure, on the shelf by the window.' '**I haven't even got pierced ears**.' Mia went and sat on the swing. It was warm in the sun and she swung gently, watching the birds in the hedge. She got off the swing and tiptoed across to the hedge. Sure enough, right in the middle of the hedge was a nest. And, what was that, **sparkling** in the straw and twigs? Mia reached in carefully and lifted it out. 'Brilliant! I'll get my Barbie now,' she said to herself as she ran **back into the house**.

What was Mia's problem? How do you know? How did she sort it out?

Story 6

Jess was going to the zoo with Nanna and Gramps. She picked up **Blob**. Blob was a rabbit made of soft fabric and Jess took him everywhere. Jess and Blob got into the back of Gramps's car. The first animal they looked at was the lion. He paced up and down, staring through the glass, blinking slowly. Then they went to find the gorillas. Today there were two baby ones chasing each other round the island and throwing sticks at each other. Jess got as close to the babies as she could. Then something awful happened. **One minute she had Blob in her hand and then, splash!** She turned to Nanna and started to cry. 'Don't worry, Jess,' said Nanna. '**We'll get it back**.' 'But I'm not sure how,' she muttered to Gramps. Just then the mother gorilla came over to the edge of the water. She bent down, reached into the reeds and **pulled something out**. And the most amazing thing happened. She looked at Jess and **threw it**, across the stream and on to the path where Jess was standing.

What was Jess's problem? How did it get sorted out? How do you know?

Level 2

Story 1

Emmie had a favourite jumper. It had blue and yellow stripes and her Nan had knitted it. She wore it every day, until Mum said, 'You've got to let me wash the jumper, Emmie: it's filthy!' Emmie grumbled a bit and then took it off. Mum put it in the washing machine and switched on the wash. Emmie went into the garden to play on the trampoline. When she came back in, Mum was pulling the washing out of the machine. 'Oh dear,' she said. She was holding up Emmie's favourite jumper. It still had blue and yellow stripes. Emmie looked very sad. 'But it's my bestist thing.' She started to cry. Mum said, 'Emmie. I'm soooo sorry, **I put the wash on too hot**. Maybe Nan could make you another.' Suddenly Emmie looked happy again. 'I know,' she said. 'I could give it to **Ted** – he hasn't even got a jumper!' She ran upstairs and grabbed the teddy off her bed.

What was the problem with Emmie's jumper? How did it get sorted out? How do you know?

Story 2

Matt got out of the car. He opened the back door and picked up his kit. They had cleared a path through the snow so he could at least walk up to the house. The woman who had phoned was standing on the doorstep looking worried. 'He's upstairs,' she said. Matt walked into the dark little kitchen. She followed Matt up the narrow staircase and into the room. There was a ladder leading up to the loft. A man lay on the floor at the bottom of the ladder. His face was a grey colour and his eyes were shut. 'Is he going to be OK?' asked Carrie, looking worried. **Matt knelt down** beside him and gently took hold of his wrist. Then he took his phone out of the bag. 'Hi, Matt Clark. I'm at 46 Canary Gardens. **Chap's had a fall, can you come straight away?**' Then he looked at Carrie and said, '**Don't worry, we'll soon get him sorted**.'

What did Matt have to sort out? How did it get sorted out? How do you know?

Story 3

It was playtime. Sam and his friends rushed outside to be first on the new pirate ship. It had come on a huge lorry the day before. It was as tall as a climbing frame and painted red, blue and green. On the top was a flag with a skull and crossbones. Sam, Joe and Ben couldn't wait to climb on board and pretend to be real pirates. Ben got there first and zoomed straight to the top of the mast. Sam clambered on to the deck part and pretended he was looking through a telescope. Then he explored the inside of the ship. It had round windows called portholes. Sam looked through them and waved to Joe who was leaning over the side above him. 'Come up here,' said Joe. 'It's brilliant!' Sam decided it would be fun to get **through the porthole**, so he stuck his head and arms through and pulled. He pulled and pulled, but **nothing happened**. He decided to go back the way he had come. Still **nothing happened**. Sam started to feel scared. 'Joe,' he called. 'Joe, help: something's gone wrong!'

What was Sam's problem? How did it get sorted out? How do you know?

Story 4

Sanjay and Mina went to the beach with their dad. Dad stuck the **umbrella in the sand**. Then he lay down on the **red and white blow-up bed**, put on his sunglasses and went to sleep. Sanjay and Mina decided to make a huge sandcastle. They dug and dug, piling up the sand into a great big dome. Mina decorated it with shells. Sanjay dug a trench all the way round it. Water flooded into the trench round the castle, turning it into a moat. The two children made little boats out of bits of driftwood to float in the moat. It was a hot afternoon. Mina said, 'Let's ask Dad for an ice cream.' They looked up, to where Dad had been sunbathing. The **umbrella** was still there, but there was water all round it. Dad wasn't there! Sanjay and Mina looked around. Then they saw something floating in the sea! **Something red and white.**

What was Dad's problem? How did it get sorted out? How do you know?

Story 5

Wendy the Witch lived in a little pink house. She had a cat called Tumble and a hen called Mrs Egg. On Tuesday Wendy went to the village shop to get her newspaper, *The Daily Spell*, and some milk. On the way to the shop she stopped to talk to Walter Wizard, who was in his garden planting giant bean seeds. When she got to the shop, she picked up the paper and the milk. She was feeling quite hungry, so she decided to have a treat. 'Mmmm, chocolate doughnuts!' she said to herself, taking a bag off the shelf. But, oh dear, when she reached in her bag for her **purse, it wasn't there**! 'Oh no. I must have left it at home!' said Wendy to Miss Hoblin, who ran the shop. Just then, Tumble walked into the shop, carrying **something** in his mouth. Something **long and thin**. 'Well done, Tums,' said Wendy, taking it out of his mouth and saying, '**Abracadabra**,' as she waved it around.

What was Wendy's problem? How did it get sorted out? How do you know?

Story 6

Alisha was really worried about the party. The **party** was that night and she wanted to look her best. It was bad enough that Samantha Higgins was going to be there. Samantha's parents were rich and bought her just about anything she wanted. And Samantha loved to show off and make other girls feel bad. Alisha stood and looked in the shop window for ages. There were such beautiful things in it! There was a **long red one with frilly sleeves**, and a pretty **blue one with stars** on it. 'I bet they are really expensive,' she thought. Then she saw the time. Help! The bus went in half an hour. This was her last chance. She pushed the door open and stepped inside.

What was Alisha's problem? How did it get sorted out? How do you know?

Level 3

Story 1

Simon really hated this job. The puppy was a champion wriggler, and in the struggle you usually got soaked. Sometimes Topsy nipped your fingers too. 'She really must be done today,' Dad said. 'She's muddy and smelly. And it's your turn, Simon.' With a sigh, Simon began to collect the things he needed. Then he went to fetch the puppy, but of course she had disappeared – she knew what was going to happen. Simon thought he knew where to look, and he went quietly out to the garden shed. Sure enough, there was Topsy, looking very unhappy, with her tail between her legs.

What was Simon's problem? How do you know? How do you think he sorted it out?

Story 2

Nikki followed the others outside. She went and stood by the wall, and munched her apple. It was quite warm in the sunshine. One group was playing tag on the grass. Others were skipping or kicking a ball around. Everyone seemed to have someone to play with. Suddenly something whizzed over her head and landed on the other side of the wall, right where Nikki was standing. She bent down and picked it up. A few seconds later she heard the sound of sobbing. 'Why did he do that? It's my best one,' cried the voice. 'My mum will be mad if I don't take it home.' The voice was coming nearer. Then Nikki saw the girl who was crying. Her two friends had their arms round her shoulders. Nikki beckoned to them.

What was Nikki's problem? How did she sort it out? How do you know?

Story 3

Mrs Sims worked fast as she sat in her chair by the window. She hoped she would get it finished in time for Billie's birthday next week. She still had the other sleeve to do and then it would need sewing together. A slight noise in the corner near the bookcase made her look up. 'Oh no,' she thought. 'I hope it hasn't got in again.' She kept looking nervously towards the little hole in the skirting board. At the same time she tucked her feet up so they weren't touching the floor. A few minutes later there was a knock on the window. Mrs Sims could see Clare from next door, mouthing something to her that she couldn't quite hear. 'Seen your what, dear?' said Mrs Sims as she opened the window.

What was Clare's problem? How do you know? How do you think she sorted it out?

Story 4

Joanna turned on the bath. She poured in some bath oil and fetched a big fluffy towel from the cupboard. Just then her phone rang. It was her best friend, Mina, calling from New York! Mina was on holiday in the United States and Joanna couldn't wait to hear all about her adventures. Downstairs Joanna's uncle Bob was watching a wildlife programme on TV. It was all about whales. Suddenly Bob realised that the sloshing, dripping noise wasn't coming from the TV.

What was Joanna's problem? How do you know? How did it get sorted out?

Story 5

Grace was very, very upset. She couldn't find Tig anywhere. Tig was her toy hedgehog and he went everywhere with her. Mum hunted all over the house and went and looked in the car. Grace didn't want her lunch. She didn't even want to watch her favourite TV programme. She just wanted Tig. A bit later Auntie Flo knocked on the door. Auntie Flo had just bought a puppy. He raced around the house, knocking things over. Grace was a bit scared of him. 'Maybe he could go out in the garden,' suggested Mum. Scamp ran round the garden, sniffing things. Suddenly he wriggled under a big bush. A few seconds later he reappeared with something in his mouth.

What was Grace's problem? How do you know? How did it get sorted out?

Story 6

Jo and Josh were on holiday at the seaside. So far it had rained every day, but at last today was warm and sunny. In the afternoon they walked along the seafront to the Crazy Golf course at the other end. About halfway along there were some benches and a little shop selling ice creams. 'Can we have an ice cream, Dad? Pleeeeeese!' Josh chose a chocolate one and Jo had strawberry. Dad had a double coffee one. They sat down and watched the boats and the surfers. Two large seagulls were searching the pavement for scraps of sandwich. 'Look, out there,' said Dad, pointing out to sea. 'There's a huge ship!' Just then Dad gasped in surprise. The cone in his hand was empty!

What was Dad's problem? How do you know? How did he sort it out?

Level 4

Story 1

'It's spurting straight up in the air and the whole path is flooded. I don't know where to turn it off!'

What is the problem? How do you know? How can it be fixed?

Story 2

She hung a star on the very top and stood back to admire it. 'Time to turn them on,' she said to herself, reaching down to the switch. A 'Pop!' Then complete darkness.

What was the problem? How do you know? How can it be fixed?

Story 3

Meg looked at her husband. The carousel had stopped turning. There were no more bags on it and the other tourists were making their way towards the exit.

What was Meg's problem? How do you know? How could it be fixed?

Story 4

'Don't worry Billy,' said Granny. 'I've saved the last one for you.' She opened the box and they both stared. Empty! Granny didn't notice Suki the dog licking his chops by the fire. Then she remembered the MegaMilk Selection box from Wendy in the office.

What was Granny's problem? How do you know? How could it be fixed?

Story 5

She looked at her watch. It had been on for 20 minutes. That's what it said on the packet: *'Leave on for 20 minutes; then rinse till the water is clear.'* Later she looked with horror in the bathroom mirror. 'It's *green!*' she cried.

What was the problem? How do you know? How can it be fixed?

Story 6

Jan had just changed for the party. She came down to answer the door. Robbins the dog came out of the dining room licking his lips. Jan peeped round the dining room door. Disaster! A broken plate, some crumbs and the candles, scattered across the floor.

What was Jan's problem? How do you know? How do you think she could fix it?

Story 7

Mrs Spin had just finished hanging the washing on the line. As she turned to go back into the house, she heard a 'Ping!' 'Oh no,' she said as she saw it all on the ground and in the flowerbeds.

What was Mrs Spin's problem? How do you know? How do you think she could fix it?

Story 8

'Look what I've got for Mum's birthday,' said Hattie. Ali looked at the box of Spring Flowers bath essence and bath oil, and sighed. Now what was she going to do? Mum wouldn't want two the same.

What was Ali's problem? How do you know? How do you think she could fix it?

Story 9

Marley was going to feed Miss Rich's cat. He walked up the road to Olive Cottage, but just as he got to the gate his phone rang. As he reached in his pocket to get the phone out, Miss Rich's key slipped out of his hand. 'Oh, help,' said Marley, looking at the metal drain cover.

What was Marley's problem? How do you know? How do you think he could fix it?

Story 10

Gran took Jamie to the bus stop. 'It's just three stops,' she said. 'If you see the town hall you've gone too far.' Jamie got on the bus and started to play with his Nintendo. It was a really good game, and the next time he looked up the bus was stopping. Outside he could see the town hall.

What was Jamie's problem? How do you know? How do you think he would fix it?

Story 11

Shania walked as fast as she could. Her sister had told her to get the Number 84 from the bus station. The last one went at 8.30 and it was already 8.25. As she turned the corner into the bus station, a bus left and Shania thought, 'What now?'

What was Shania's problem? How do you know? How do you think she would fix it?

Story 12

Robbie loved Tuesdays because it was Swimming. After break he picked up his swimming bag and went across to the changing rooms. Today he hoped he would be able to go underwater. He pulled his kit out of the swimming bag and looked in horror at the pink frilly bathing costume!

What was Robbie's problem? How do you know? How do you think he would fix it?

Cause - effect

Level 1

Find the clues that tell you WHY SOMETHING HAPPENED, or why something might be going to happen.

Here is an example. The clues are in bold type.

Jade was just **running her bath** when the **phone rang**. 'It's for you,' her mum called up the stairs. **Jade** wrapped herself in a towel, **ran downstairs** and **picked up the phone**. It was her best friend, saying the new film they wanted to see was opening in two days' time. They fixed to meet at their favourite pasta restaurant, and have a meal there before the film. They **started talking about the film**, and wondering how it ended. There were several big stars in it. Suddenly there was a cry from the kitchen. 'For heaven's sake!' **Mum was shouting**. 'There's **water trickling through the kitchen ceiling**.' Jade banged down the phone and rushed into the kitchen. Now the **water was pouring down**. She suddenly **realised what had happened**.

Why was there water in the kitchen? How do you know?

- *Jade was running her bath when the phone rang*
- *She ran downstairs to the phone*
- *She spent a long time arranging to meet her friend and discussing the film*
- *Water started coming through the ceiling*
- *Jade had forgotten to turn her bath off*

Story 1

Sam **stared in horror at the rabbit hutch**. The **door** was **swinging open**, and Fluffy the **rabbit** was **nowhere to be seen**. **Sam** was the **only person who looked after Fluffy**, and he always **locked the door** after feeding him. Sam **felt in his pockets**. The **key was there**! Sam ran into the kitchen, calling his mum. 'Mum, Fluffy has escaped. Come and help!' Mum was good in emergencies like this. She followed Sam into the garden, carrying some carrot and some bits of toast, which Fluffy loved. It wasn't long before there was a rustling in the flowerbed and the rabbit's face peered out. When he was safely **back in his hutch**, Sam **locked the hutch door** with extra care, and **hung the key on the hook where it** was meant to be. He promised himself he **would never forget again**.

Why did Fluffy escape? How do you know?

Story 2

Ryan lay on the sofa, with his **leg up on the cushions**. The **plaster on his leg** was covered in squiggly writing, where his friends had put their names on it. The **plaste**r had **been on for six weeks**, and he was due to go to the **hospital the next day to have it taken off**. Then he would be given a pair of crutches and be allowed to walk about, as long as he went carefully. Out of the window he could see where the last of the **snow was melting**. The ducks were swimming on the pond again, so the ice **must have melted** too. He had been doing so well until **he had tried to go too fast** and **crashed into** the bank. It looked as if they would have to **wait till the next winter** for a chance to **go skating again**.

Why was Ryan's leg in plaster? How do you know?

Story 3

Beth **woke up feeling awful**. Her **throat was sore**, her **eyes itched** and **she felt really hot**. She absolutely could not go to school, she thought, whatever Mum said. She went downstairs and told her mum how she felt. 'Can you manage **a bit of breakfast**?' Mum asked. Beth **started on a bowl of cereal**, but after two mouthfuls she **didn't want any more**. '**You really must be ill**,' **Mum said.** 'Come on back upstairs, and **I'll take your temperature**.' It was quite high. Mum took another look at Beth. 'Aha,' she said. 'I **think I know what's the matter. Amy went down with chickenpox** after her **birthday party**, didn't she? Take a look at your face in the mirror.' When Beth looked, she could see the **beginnings of a splodgy rash**.

Why was Beth ill? How do you know?

Story 4

It was fun to be home after the holiday. Mum went straight into the kitchen to make cups of tea and coffee. 'There's a **funny smell in here**,' she said, sniffing. 'Oh heavens, and there's a huge **puddle by the freezer**.' Everyone came into the kitchen. 'Mind where you tread,' Mum said. 'I don't want you trampling wet feet all over the house.' She threw some old towels down to mop up the flood, and **went cautiously** over **to the freezer**. As soon as **she opened it, the smell got much worse**. Mum held her nose as she looked inside. 'Oh no,' she wailed. '**Everything has defrosted** and **most of it** looks as if it **has gone bad**.' Dad was looking dreadfully guilty. 'I must have **done that plug as well** by mistake **when I switched off the washing machine**,' he said.

Why was the freezer not working? How do you know?

Story 5

Ben woke in the morning wondering if he had actually slept at all with the **noise of the wind**. He ran to look out of the window. A huge branch off the old beech tree **lay across the lawn**, and the tallest **flowers** in the flowerbed were all **lying flat** on the ground. Ben quickly pulled on some clothes and ran downstairs. His **dad** was **trying to** make a **phone** call, but **didn't seem to be getting through**. It was rather dark in the kitchen and Ben **pressed the light switch**, but **no light came on**. 'What's going on?' Ben asked his mum. '**No electricity and no phone**,' she said. 'There may be no school either.' It turned out that **school was shut**, because there were **trees down all over the road**. He had a great day helping Dad saw up the beech branch and stack the logs in the shed.

Why had all these things happened? How do you know?

Story 6

Poppy felt very miserable. She **sat at her desk**, and **out of the window** she **could see** all her **friends having fun in the playground**. She looked at the sheet of paper in front of her, with the list of **spellings she should have learnt for homework** the night before. How **she wished** now **she hadn't watched TV instead!** She had meant to learn them this morning, but she had **only had a quick look at them. Mr Hutchins had been really cross**. Now he was wandering around the classroom, keeping a beady eye on Poppy all the time. Poppy picked up the list with a sigh, and tried to concentrate, but the sound of laughter and shouting from the playground kept distracting her. Once, her friend Jasmine came up to the window and made a face at her through the glass.

Why was Poppy the only child in the classroom? How do you know?

Level 2

Story 1

That January **it rained and rained and rained. Adam's house was** quite **near the river**; in fact the river was just across the road. As the rain went on falling, they could **see the river rising** until it was **nearly at the top of the bank**. The **weather forecast** on the radio **talked about more rain** in the next few days, heavier than usual. Adam's **dad rang up to get sandbags** to put by the door. 'And we'd **better get the carpets up**, and **take the best furniture upstairs**,' he said. Adam helped as they started to shift stuff up into the bedrooms.

Why did they get the carpets up and take the best furniture upstairs? How do you know?

Story 2

Rita **got into the car beside the examiner**. Now that the time had actually come **for her test**, she was really nervous. She *must* remember the things her instructor had told her – use the **indicator**, and **look in the mirror** to see what's behind you. She **pulled out into the road**. A **car swerved to overtake her**, and **hooted his horn**. The examiner made a **note** on his pad. She drove carefully, keeping an eye on her speed. 'Turn right' at the next lights,' said the examiner. Rita started to move over **into the right hand lane**. There was **another furious hoot from a car** that was **coming right up behind her**. **Rita didn't even know it was there!** She realised **she was going to fail the test**.

Why did Rita fail her driving test? How do you know?

Story 3

Ashok **spotted the wallet** lying in the gutter. He nearly left it there, as it was soaking wet and muddy and looked as if it had been there for ages. Then he changed his mind, and **went back for it**. When he looked inside, he was amazed to find **there were several £10 notes in it**. Ashok **took it to the** nearby **police station** and handed it in. The policeman on duty took Ashok's name and address, and said thank you. Three weeks **later a letter came through the post** for Ashok. **Inside was a £20 note**, and a letter from someone called Mrs Burson. The letter said Ashok was a good, honest boy and to buy himself something nice with the money.

Why did Ashok get a letter with £20 in it? How do you know?

Story 4

Jacob **got into the lift**, clutching his parcels and an umbrella. He was worried that he was late meeting his mates. They had **arranged to meet on the sixth floor** of the shop, **where the cafe was**. Jacob quickly **pressed the top button**. The lift doors slid shut, the lift gave a wheeze and began to go up. When the doors opened again, Jacob got out and found himself **stepping out on to the roof**! There was a great view, but no sign of the cafe. Jacob hurried back to the lift, and took a careful look at the floor numbers. Aha! The **top button was Number 7**. What a silly mistake, he thought to himself, as he took the lift back down a floor.

Why did Jacob find himself on the wrong floor? How do you know?

Story 5

On Boxing Day Mum spent ages making a lovely **lunch out of the left-over turkey**. It had all sorts of things in it, and smelt really good. 'I **need this to cool down** before I can put it in the fridge,' she said to Dad. 'Can you open this window a bit? The cold air will do the trick.' Dad **pushed the window up a few inches**, and Mum **put the big dish beside it**. 'That's sorted supper out,' she said, 'I'm going to sit down and put my feet up for a few minutes.' When Mum went back into the kitchen **an hour later**, **half her lovely turkey pie was gone**. Next door's **dog**, the one with the long, thin, pointy nose, **was legging it** across the back garden.

Why was Mum's turkey dish half gone? How do you know?

Story 6

The washing machine had broken down, so **Nan** had kindly offered to do **the family wash** for them. Mohammed lugged the basket to Nan's house three doors down the street. He watched **as Nan put the things in the machine** and piled **some of her own tea cloths and towels in as well**. Then she and Mohammed sat down for a drink and a biscuit. Nan had the best biscuits in the world. **When Nan took the washing out** of the machine, she gave a little cry. **Everything was bright yellow**! Luckily Mum thought it was funny. 'Poor Nan,' she said. 'She's a bit forgetful these days. She **must have put some dusters in** with the clothes.'

Why did all the clothes turn yellow? How do you know?

Level 3

Story 1

It was the night of Bethany's eighteenth birthday party. At six o'clock people started to arrive. More and more came, and some of them Bethany didn't know at all. She tried to stop them, but they just went on crowding in. Beth's father was absolutely furious. That Facebook message had been a big mistake.

Why were strangers coming to Bethany's party? How do you know?

Story 2

Ben got his bike out and set off to the shop. He was going to get his lottery ticket, and buy some glue for the model he was making. There was some broken glass on the road, and Ben cycled carefully round to try to avoid it. When he came out of the shop, he was upset to find his tyre was flat.

Why did Ben have a flat tyre? How do you know?

Story 3

Aneena went into the conservatory to do her homework. She sat down and opened a book; then something caught her eye. All Grandpa's beloved geraniums were drooping sadly. The pots looked bone dry. She realised she had forgotten the promise she had made Grandpa when he went on holiday.

Why were Grandpa's flowers drooping? How do you know?

Story 4

The teacher came into the classroom and stopped in amazement. She began to smile and then to laugh, and soon there were tears of happiness in her eyes. The children's hard work putting up the balloons, and getting the cake, and making the '40th birthday' banner had all been worthwhile.

Why was the teacher so happy? How do you know?

Story 5

Dad stopped outside the front door. The glass in the door was broken. Inside he found Mum's jewellery box lying on the floor of the living room, smashed and empty. A clock had gone too, and the DVD recorder. Furious and upset, Dad reached for his mobile and dialled 999.

Why did Dad phone the police? How do you know?

Story 6

Auntie Ritala banged on the door. 'Gran's not well!' she shouted to Mum. 'She's a funny colour and she won't wake up. My phone's not working – can I use yours?' Five minutes later Sita was watching out of the window as an ambulance raced up the street, bells clanging and lights flashing.

Why was an ambulance coming? How do you know?

Level 4

Story 1

'Drat that Muffin,' Mum muttered to herself crossly, as she brushed the pawmarks off the cushions and threw the half-chewed bone into the waste paper basket.

Why were there pawmarks and a bone on the sofa? How do you know?

Story 2

Annie saw the remains of the fish pie on the floor, and Mojo's tail disappearing out of the door and up the apple tree.

Why was the fish pie on the floor? How do you know?

Story 3

'Oh no,' wailed Bess. 'Mr Black will be so cross. It was PE we were late for last week too.'

Why was Bess upset? How do you know?

Story 4

Suddenly the train went dark for a minute, and then they were out in the sunshine again.

Why did the train go dark for a minute? How do you know?

Story 5

Rover took one look at the bucket of water and the sponge, and vanished down the back steps.

Why did Rover run away? How do you know?

Story 6

On the other side of the ford was a big sign reading 'Test your brakes'. Mum tried, but nothing happened.

Why didn't Mum's brakes work? How do you know?

Story 7

'That's the last time I'll lend my brother my car,' Bob said furiously to himself, as he dabbed paint on the latest set of scratches.

Why wouldn't Bob lend his brother his car again? How do you know?

Story 8

Johnnie came in from his long day by the river, and stowed his rod and net in the hall. 'Any luck?' called his dad. Johnnie shouted triumphantly, 'Six!'

What was Johnnie so pleased about? How do you know?

Story 9

When Alice looked out of the window, there was just a heap of snow where the snowman had been and water was dripping off the eaves.

Why was there water dripping off the eaves? How do you know?

Story 10

As Jenny opened her eyes and stared muzzily at the brand new plaster on her arm, the memory of that last go at the skatepark came flooding back.

Why did Jenny have a plaster on her arm? How do you know?

Story 11

Feeling a little bit sick, Damian hid the empty chocolate box in the waste paper basket.

Why did Damian feel sick? How do you know?

Story 12

The man climbed his ladder to the first window, carrying a heavy pot of paint. 'I'm afraid it's going to be a big job after 20 years or more,' said Dad.

Why did the man climb up the ladder? How do you know?

Time

Level 1

Find the clues that tell you WHEN something happened/will happen.

Clues might be about:

- The time of day

- The time of year

- The day or month

- A special day or festival

- The past or the future

- Times when things keep happening

Here is an example. The clues are in bold type.

George got out of bed, and then wished he hadn't – his **bedroom felt so cold**. There was a sort of **white light everywhere**. He went to the window, his bare feet feeling icy on the floor. Out of the window the garden looked quite different from usual. The **ground was white**, and there was a **white covering on the branches** of the trees, the **top of the car** and the **other cars** in the street. There were already **people out** in the street **with shovels**, **clearing paths** from their front doors to the pavement. George reached for his clothes, a **thick jumper** and some **woolly socks**. He wondered if with luck **school might be closed**. Pity there were no hills in the town, or they **could have gone tobogganing**.

What time of year was it? How do you know?

- *It was icy cold*

- *There was white stuff on the ground and on the branches of the trees*

- *People were shovelling to clear pathways*

- *School might be closed*

- *It was the sort of weather for tobogganing*

- *It must have been winter*

Story 1

Millie **finished her cornflakes**. She had finished all the interesting cereals the day before. She started the daily **hunt to find her school bag** and her **PE things** – she never remembered to put them ready before she went to bed. While she was searching around, the usual mad panic started. Her little **brother started crying** because he **didn't want to go to nursery**, her big sister was grumbling about something, and Dad was yelling that **it was getting late**, and to **hurry up** or the **girls would miss their bus**. Millie spotted her trainers in a corner, stuffed them into her bag, **blew a kiss to her mum**, and **set off** with Laura **to catch the school bus**.

What time of day was it? How do you know?

Story 2

Joe's class at school were doing a project on space, and there had also been a **programme** on TV about the **stars**. Joe was really interested. He had **a book called** *Star Stories*, and he wanted to go **outside in the dark** to see for himself. Would he **be able to spot the stars** he had been told about? He **took a torch** and his book, and went down the garden as far as he could, where the **lights from the street** didn't stop him from seeing the sky clearly. He **shone his torch** on the first picture. It was **the Plough (or the Great Bear)**. He tipped his head back to look at the sky, and he thought he had found it. The trouble was, he really needed to be able to look at the picture and the sky at the same time!

What time of day was it? How do you know?

Story 3

Everyone had been helping to **build the huge pile of logs and twigs**, and now it was about three metres high. Some people had even got rid of old chairs and bits of broken furniture and had piled them on too. The **figure, made of broomsticks** for arms and a **football for a head**, was propped **on the very top**. It was beginning to get dark, and it was **time for the fire to be lit**. Elinor and Kirsty had a **packet of sparklers** each. They were **wrapped up in their warmest clothes**, and set off with the family and their friends to see the fun. The **fire was lit**, and began to burn brightly. Then the first **firework shot up into the sky**, and another one burst into showers of tiny stars. There were **burgers to eat**, cooked on a barbecue.

What special day in the year was it? How do you know?

Story 4

Nan seemed very excited when she came in from the garden. 'I can just see **some snowdrops coming up**,' she said. 'Come and look.' The children went with her, but couldn't really see what the fuss was about. There were just some **little green shoots poking up** above the ground. 'And look over there,' said Nan. A big **black bird had flown into a tree**, **carrying a piece of straw** in its beak. 'The first **birds** are thinking about **building their nests**,' said Nan. 'The rooks are always the first, but they're a bit too early this year. There could be **some cold weather to come still**. But it does mean the **long dark days are nearly over**. I always **love this time of year**.' 'Old people do get worked up about the weirdest things,' said Amy as they went back into the house.

What time of year was it? How do you know?

Story 5

Alex's little sister, **Alice, was thrilled**. She was only two, so she had no idea what it was all about, but she was enjoying the bustle and all the **new things** that **were happening**. She tried to help when Alex and his **dad dragged the tree into the house**, but she got dreadfully in the way. She **loved hanging** the **decorations on the tree**, and especially **draping the tinsel** all **over the branches**. When **Alex switched on the fairy lights**, Alice screamed with excitement. Alex **helped her** to **hang up her stocking** on the **end of her bunk bed**, and tried to explain to her that it **would be full of presents** in the morning, but she didn't really understand. She just wanted to put the big stocking on her head for a hat. Dad said he would hang it up properly when Alice was asleep.

What special day in the year was it? How do you know?

Story 6

Nidal thought this was the **best day of the week. No school**, and **football** as usual **in the afternoon**. He got dressed in his team kit, all except the boots, which Mum didn't let him wear in the house. After breakfast, he went round to his **best friend's house** and they **played on their iPods** for a bit. **After lunch**, four of the team met and **rode their bikes down to the football pitch**. The coach met them as they walked over from the bike park. 'The team you're playing today are really great,' he said. 'You'll have to be on top form if you're going to beat them. Do your best. You've got **tomorrow to have a rest** and recover in!' Nidal saw his family arrive to watch, and gave them a wave. Then the **teams took up positions on the pitch, and the coach blew his whistle**.

What day of the week was it? How do you know?

Level 2

Story 1

The wind was **blowing a gale**. In the park the **leaves were tumbling off the trees** and blowing into big drifts on the ground. **They** were **beautiful colours**: red and orange and yellow. Someone's dad said it was good luck to catch a leaf as it was falling, before it touched the ground, and you should catch twelve, one for each month of the year. The children tried to catch some, and got a few, but it was harder than it looked. It was **starting to get dark earlier each day now**, so **by teatime** they **couldn't see well enough** to go on playing. Still nobody had caught twelve leaves.

What season of the year was it? How do you know?

Story 2

The pictures in the book showed a family **sitting outside a cave**. They were **not wearing clothes, just animal skins**. The **man** in the picture **had a spear** in his hand. The **woman** was **cooking something over a fire**. It looked like a lump of meat, and it was **stuck on a pointed stick**, **not** put in a **cooking pot**. Among the trees in the distance were **strange-looking animals**, a bit like cows but not quite the same. Nearby were other people, also dressed in skins. They all had wild, long hair and looked very fierce.

Was this story about past times, the present or the future? How do you know?

Story 3

Mum gave Ellie a kiss, **turned the light off**, and **shut the bedroom door**. Ellie waited until she heard **Mum's footsteps going down the stairs**, and the **landing light went out**. Quietly she pulled her iPod out from **under the covers** where she had hidden it, and switched it on. She was halfway through a really good game and was longing to see if she could manage to get to the end of the level.

What time of day was it? How do you know?

Story 4

Sue was going through her cupboard, pulling out clothes and flinging them on her bed. 'I haven't got a thing to wear in this **boiling weather**,' she said to her friend Jackie, who was sitting on the bed, watching. 'Unless I **spend all day in a swimsuit**, the only thing I bought last year, so it should still be all right.' 'Not a bad idea, though,' said Jackie. 'We could go to the Leisure Centre and **have a swim**.'

What time of year was it? How do you know?

Story 5

Aunt May had been staying with the family. She started the morning in a bit of a bad mood. 'I always **hate this day**,' she said '**After a lovely** lazy **weekend**, it's really **hard to go back to the office**.' Dad wasn't very sympathetic. 'Cheer up!' he said. 'It'll **soon be** the end of another week and **a weekend again**.' Aunt May made a face at him. 'Just because YOU don't have to go to work today,' she said.

What day of the week was it? How do you know?

Story 6

The big silver shuttle-ship glided in to land. The **passengers floated out** using their **flight backpacks**, and disappeared in all directions into the **intergalactic transit station**. Now it was William and his family's turn. They went up the steps of the shuttle-ship in the **old fashioned way, on their feet**. Inside the ship they were locked into their **individual sealed compartments**, which were padded to avoid injury as they floated in the **weightless atmosphere**. A high humming noise began, and the ship began its **supersonic journey** to the **asteroid halfway station**.

Is this story about the past, the present, or the future? How do you know?

Level 3

Story 1

The children put their things in their school bags, and got their coats off their usual pegs. The name labels by the pegs had already been taken down, and new names were being put up. They all went up to Mr Forbes and said goodbye. 'I know you think I've given you a hard time,' Mr Forbes said with a grin. 'Just wait till you see what Mr Gibson's like! You'll wish you were back in Year 5!'

What special day was it? How do you know?

Story 2

Robbie looked at his watch. Only five minutes to go. The first half of the morning always seemed to drag on Thursdays. That was probably because the first lesson was numeracy, and Robbie hated numeracy, and the second one was Humanities with Mr Hayward, who nearly managed to send them all to sleep. Just then the bell rang, and the class jumped to their feet and made for the door.

What part of the day was it? How do you know?

Story 3

Mum sat down by the children's beds, and took out the book. They were just getting to the exciting bit. She put on her spooky voice and began: 'It was a pitch black night. From time to time an owl hooted, and a fox gave its eerie bark. The grandfather clock began to strike – bong, bong – and as the last of the twelve bongs sounded, the witch sprang out of the cupboard with a shriek.'

What time was it in the story? How do you know?

Story 4

Everything went wrong for Peter that morning. First he couldn't find his football boots, then his homework had vanished, and then there was none of his favourite cereal. He dithered so long about what to eat that Mum said he would miss the bus. The Number 11 was always at the stop at exactly 8 o'clock, and when Peter finally ran out of the door he knew he was in trouble. Sure enough, as he panted up to the bus stop, he saw the back of the bus disappearing round the corner.

What time was it when Peter got to the bus stop? How do you know?

Story 5

The reporter from the local newspaper was coming to write a piece about the play. Damien did so hope that the reporter would say something nice about his sword fight in the first scene. The rehearsal went well, and the reporter said how much he had enjoyed it . But the paper next morning was disappointing. There was nothing about the sword fight, and in fact nothing about the first two scenes. It didn't sound as if the reporter had got the hang of the story at all.

When did the reporter get to the rehearsal? How do you know?

Story 6

There was a new cook in the school kitchen. He made the most fantastic Yorkshire puddings. They were so popular, there were never enough. Twice now Darrell had missed out, and had to make do without his Yorkshire. He made up his mind this was not going to happen again. The next time there was a roast dinner Darrell kept his eye on the clock. As dinner time got closer, he sat on the edge of his chair, ready to make a dash for the queue.

Did Darrell plan to be before or after everyone else getting to the canteen? How do you know?

Level 4

Story 1

When Amelia woke, she could just see the beginnings of a glimmer of light in the sky, and wondered if she should get up yet.

What time of day was it? How do you know?

Story 2

When the older children came down to breakfast, Joanne already had chocolate smeared all over her face, and pieces of chocolate eggshell on her plate.

What special day was it? How do you know?

Story 3

As Gemma tore open the first of her cards, a badge with a big number 6 fell out, and Gemma pinned it carefully on to the front of her T-shirt.

What special day was it? How do you know?

Story 4

Josh and Ed put on their skull masks, grabbed a torch and a bag for the sweets, and set off into the dark.

What special day was it? How do you know?

Story 5

That Saturday Sadeep came home on his bike from the outdoor pool, and hung his swimming trunks out to dry. He was sad to think that his next weekly swimming lesson was a whole six days away.

What time of year was it? How do you know?

Story 6

Will gave a last loving polish to his motorbike as the clock struck ten. It did seem a bit of a waste to get it looking so good when the race was due to start in half an hour, and it would be covered in mud again.

What was the race? How do you know?

Story 7

'Thank heavens for the end of another week,' said the head teacher, as he signalled the close of the staff meeting.

What day of the week was it? How do you know?

Story 8

'I can't get away till one,' said Dad on the phone, 'but it only takes me about ten minutes to walk.'

What time would Dad meet his friend? How do you know? How was he going to get there?

Story 9

Beth feared she was in for yet another detention as she handed in her unfinished work.

Had Beth had detention before? How do you know? Why was she being given detention?

Story 10

'This is the last lot on your present prescription,' said the chemist, handing over the packet of pills to Grandma, 'so don't forget to renew it.'

Would Grandma need more pills in future? How do you know? What would she have to do?

Story 11

'Not you again!' said the policeman, marching the two boys and their football off the forbidden grass. 'Can't you see the sign?'

What had the boys been doing? Had they been caught before? How do you know? How could they know it wasn't allowed?

Story 12

Leah gazed around the beautiful little bay, thinking how often she had dreamed of coming back to here.

Had Leah been to the bay before? How do you know? Did she remember it well?

Character/feelings

Level 1

Find the clues that tell you WHAT KIND OF PERSON they are, or HOW THEY WERE FEELING.

Clues might be about:

- What the person was like

- What they felt like

Here is an example. The clues are in bold type.

Jez looked at the **list of names** on the notice board. They were all the people who had been **picked for the team**. He was sure his name would be there. He looked and looked, but couldn't see *Jeremy Hudson* anywhere. 'Nope,' he thought. '**Not picked**, again.' He pulled up the hood of his hoodie, put his hands in his pockets and walked out into the street. It wasn't far to Nan's house. When he got there, Nan was sitting in the kitchen with a mug of tea. 'Oh, Jez, love. What is it?' she said when he walked in and slumped into a chair by the fire. '**It's not fair**, Nan,' muttered Jez. 'I'm the **best goalie** they've ever had, so **why haven't I been picked**?'

How is Jez feeling? How do you know?

- *Jez played football*

- *He was looking at the list of players chosen for the team*

- *His name was not on the list*

- *He went to tell his Nan about it*

- *Jez was feeling fed up because he hadn't been chosen*

Story 1

Rose Smith lived at Number 24 Plum Street. She had lived there for a long, long time. Every day she walked down to the shop to get some milk and a newspaper. On Monday morning there was a huge lorry parked outside. Soon she heard thumping noises from next door. 'Ah-ha,' said Rose. 'Someone must be moving in at last.' She finished her cup of tea and set off for the shop as usual. That day she bought **a packet of chocolate biscuits and an extra carton of milk** as well as the paper. On her way home she met Tom Bloggins, from the pub. 'Morning Tom,' she called. 'How's Betty?' 'Not so good,' said Tom. **'I'll pop over and see her later**,' said Rose and carried on up the hill. When she got to her house, the lorry was still there. Rose took her shopping into the house. Then she took one of the **cartons of milk and the packet of biscuits** and went and knocked on the door of Number 22. **'Welcome to Plum Street**,' she said to the man who opened the door.

What sort of person was Rose? How do you know?

Story 2

It was the summer holidays and so far it had rained every day. Milly sat looking at the raindrops running down the window. She could see the trampoline at the end of the garden. Mum and Dad had given it to her for her birthday two days before. Milly was so excited when she saw it that morning. She couldn't wait to have a go, but Mum said, 'Sorry, Mil. You'll have to wait till the rain stops.' And it hadn't. Milly went up to her room. There were colouring books and craft sets and Barbies and bead-making kits. But she just **didn't want to do any of it**. What she wanted was to bounce on her trampoline and fly up towards the sky. She sat on the floor for a bit, **flicking little bits of paper** under her bed. Then she got up and went downstairs again. Still raining. **Still no chance** of going outside. She put the TV on, **but there were only programmes for little kids**. Yuk! She went back to sit by the window, watching the raindrops racing each other down the glass.

How did Milly feel? How do you know?

Story 3

Wizzo the wizard lived in Toadville. Every year all the wizards in Toadville had a special party in Toadville Hall. Everyone had to bring something to eat and a new spell to show their wizard friends. This year Wizzo was going to make a delicious Gunge Cake with frogspawn icing. He had bought a new magic wand made of fairy oak, which is a very special kind of wood with extra magic powers. He looked at the recipe for the cake. 'Uh-oh,' he said. 'It says you need five snake eggs, but I **didn't get any** when I went shopping! Oh well, maybe spiders' eggs will do.' Next he had to do the icing. The trouble was he **hadn't bought any frogspawn either** so he had to use toadspawn from his pond. On the day of the party he set off to Toadville Hall. He put his cake on the table with all the other food. 'Wizzo, show us your spell,' said the Master Wizard. Wizzo reached for his wand **but it wasn't in his bag. Or his pocket. Or anywhere.**

What kind of a wizard was Wizzo? How do you know

Story 4

My name is Billy Bell and I'm nine years old. I'm really good at sport, especially football, and I bet I'm the fastest runner in the class. Everyone wants to be my friend 'cos **I'm so cool**. My dad has a really fast car and my mum is a singer and she's famous. **I'm the boss of a gang** called The Brillos. It's hard to get into our gang 'cos **I'm really fussy about who joins**. This week a new kid came to our school. He came up to me in the playground and asked if he could join our gang. He's called Jeremy and he's got glasses and he likes reading. I told the others, 'Guess what, guys, this is Jeremy. He likes reading. **He probably reads so much that his eyes have got worn out, so he wears glasses!**' The others laughed when I said that. Jeremy didn't. 'Come on Jez, let's try your glasses, then,' I said, **pulling them off him**. He tried to snatch them back but I threw them to Floyd. Jeremy started whingeing about not being able to see, **but we just laughed**.

What sort of a boy was Billy? How do you know?

Story 5

Mina felt someone shaking her and heard her dad say, 'Come on, Mina, it's time to get up.' Mina opened her eyes. The room was dark. Outside it was still night time. Dad was dressed and there were two suitcases by the bedroom door. Then she remembered. She was suddenly wide awake. **At last the day had come**. She had been **waiting so long** for this. She got out of bed and dressed as quickly as she could. They had to leave really early, before it was properly light. Mina thought about arriving at the beach house in Spain and seeing her friend Franca again. They would be able to swim in the pool and explore the beach and hide in the pine trees. **Mina couldn't believe** it was **really going to happen today**. Dad said she had to have a proper breakfast before they left, but she didn't want anything. It seemed such a long way to the airport and such a long wait when they got there. But at last their flight was called, and **Mina's eyes were shining** as they walked up the steps to the plane.

How did Mina feel? How do you know?

Story 6

Jenna Jones was walking her dog, Frosty. It was a sunny afternoon and Jenna decided to go along the path by the canal. There were some houseboats on the canal and Jenna wondered what it would be like living on a boat. The trouble was, she couldn't swim and **she was frightened of going in the water**. Just then Jenna wondered where Frosty was. 'Frosty,' she called. 'Come on, Frosty. Here boy!' Then she saw him, charging down the hill. Some children saw the dog and one of them threw a stick into the water. **Frosty** plunged in after it, but he **couldn't get out** again because the bank was so steep. Jenna was frantic with worry. She looked around. No one in sight. What was she to do? Frosty was scrabbling at the slippery sides of the bank, but the current was pulling at him. Jenna kicked off her shoes and **slid down into the water**. Luckily her feet touched the muddy bottom of the canal, and she was able to get hold of Frosty's collar.

What sort of person was Jenna? How do you know?

Level 2

Story 1

Adam was really excited. He had been invited to Ajay's birthday treat. On the invitation it said they were going to the ice rink. Adam had **never been ice skating** before. 'Mum,' he said, 'I don't have any ice skates. What's going to happen?' Mum told him that he could hire the skates when they got there. Adam **couldn't believe that Ajay had actually asked him** to his treat. Ajay was the coolest boy in Year 4. He always had the best trainers and the latest phone. He didn't usually even talk to Adam, let alone invite him out. Adam thought about ice skating. **Probably Ajay and all his friends would be brilliant** at skating. They probably went every week. Adam looked up the ice rink on Mum's laptop. There was a video of kids doing amazing moves and spinning and even jumping. Adam **took a deep breath**. 'It'll be OK,' he told himself.

How did Adam feel about going ice skating? How do you know?

Story 2

Josh pasted the last picture into his project. It was all about what it was like being a kid in World War 2. His great-nan had been evacuated to Devon, to a great big farmhouse on Exmoor. She had some photos, just a few, in an old album. Josh's big sister, May, scanned them so he could put them into his project, and tomorrow he was going to hand it in. The next morning he gave it to Mrs Soames. On Friday it was **special Assembly** at school, the sort where parents can come. Josh's mum brought his nan, and he could see them sitting at the back. The head teacher said, 'I've got a special announcement today. **Year 4 have been doing projects** about World War 2 and we have decided that the **best project of all is Josh Simpson's**. Well done, Josh! Let's give him a clap! Josh couldn't believe it. He looked at his mum and nan, there at the back of the hall. **Their faces were smiling** and they were clapping really hard. '**Wow**,' thought Josh.

How do you think Josh felt? How do you know?

Story 3

A long time ago there was a princess called Tia who lived with the king and queen in a castle. Near the castle there was a village, and sometimes Tia would look over the walls and **watch the village children** playing. **Tia wasn't allowed** to go to the village. She had to stay in the castle gardens, **just her** and Pounce. Tia didn't go to school. She had someone called a governess whose name was Miss Fripp. Miss Fripp made Tia do Maths and Reading and Writing. But what **Tia really wanted to do was go and play** with the village children. She wanted to join in their games and sing their songs and eat jam sandwiches out of a paper bag. 'Come on, Tia,' called Miss Fripp. 'Stop looking over the wall and wasting your time, you've got spellings to do.' Tia sighed and walked slowly back to boring Miss Fripp. **It wasn't fair.**

How did Tia feel? How do you know?

Story 4

Jan, Katya and Jorgo were staying with their nan and grandpa in the country. Nan and Grandpa had a big, old house with a huge garden. Jan was nine and he was the eldest. Jorgo was seven and Katya was five. It was the beginning of the holidays and the children were excited about exploring the garden. But when they woke up the next day, it was pouring with rain. They decided to explore inside the house instead. They went right up to the attics. There were three rooms up there. The first two were full of dusty furniture and boxes. There was nothing in the third room, apart from an old rug on the floor. Jan and Katya went back into the first room and found some old puzzles in a box. Jorgo stood in the empty room on the worn old rug. Suddenly a voice said, 'Follow the light you will see in the woods and you will be rewarded.' Jorgo looked around but there was no one there. Then he heard Jan calling him. 'Jorgo, what are you doing? Have you found something interesting?' '**Nope**,' said Jorgo, '**nothing at all**.'

What sort of a boy was Jorgo? How do you know?

Story 5

Hannah's little sister was called Jemima, but everyone called her Mima. Mima had amazing hair; everyone said so. It was blonde and very curly and a bit wild. Hannah's hair was straight and brown, and not the sort of hair you would notice. '**I don't see what's so great about blonde curls, anyway**,' Hannah grumbled to herself. 'It'll probably go straight when she's bigger.' Today it was Mima's sixth birthday and she was having a party. Mum was busy icing the cake in the kitchen. Hannah asked her for a biscuit. 'Hannah, can't you see how busy I am?' said Mum. The cake was in the shape of a castle and there was a little princess to put on the top. '**When it was my birthday, she got one from the supermarket**,' grumbled Hannah. Mima was in the sitting room, surrounded by wrapping paper and cards and presents. 'Look, Han. Look what I've got! Three new Barbies to go in my new Barbie house! Come on, let's sort them all out!' '**Barbies are boring**,' muttered Hannah as she screwed up bits of torn wrapping paper and flicked them at the wall.

How was Hannah feeling? How do you know?

Story 6

Mrs Rose was a busy lady. On Mondays she **helped** at the school, listening to children reading. On Tuesdays she **took library books round to old people** who were stuck at home. She had three grandchildren and they all came to tea on Wednesdays after school. After tea she **helped** them with their homework and read them stories. Thursdays was dog walking day. Mrs Rose **took two people's dogs for walks while they were at work**. The other thing Mrs Rose liked was competitions. She was always going in for them but she never won anything. However, on Friday 13 July all that changed. Mrs Rose heard the sound of the post falling on the mat. A plain white envelope. She opened it and inside was a cheque for £10,000! Mrs Rose sat down, amazed. Then straight away she phoned her daughter. 'You know that trip to Italy Finn wanted to go on? Well, sign the paper: **he can go!**'

What kind of person was Mrs Rose? How do you know?

Level 3

Story 1

Dwayne fetched the fish food, and went to feed his guppies. When he looked into the fish tank, he could see only three of them. He tapped the sides of the tank in case one was hiding in the tunnel or under the clump of weed, but no fish came out. He sprinkled the food on top of the water, and the three guppies shot up, gulping, but still there was no sign of the fourth one. Dwayne had to go off to school, and he worried all day about what had happened to his fish. When he got home in the evening, he asked his mum to help him lift the three guppies out and empty the water. Right in the little rock tunnel lay the body of the fourth guppy.

How did Dwayne feel? How do you know?

Story 2

It was nearly dark when Barry got home from school. There were no lights on in the house , but he knew nobody else would be back yet. He put his key in the door, pushed it open, and reached for the light switch. The light didn't come on. He groped around in the hall for the door into the living room, and reached for the light switch in there. Still nothing happened. None of the lights he tried seemed to be working. There was always a big torch in the hall cupboard, so he felt his way back and opened the cupboard door. No torch. Barry stood still, wondering what to do. As he stood there, he heard something moving in the kitchen. Then the sound of shuffling footsteps started coming nearer and nearer, and he could hear someone or something breathing heavily. The hair stood up on the back of Barry's neck, his heart began to race, and he squeezed into the corner between the stairs and the cupboard. Whatever it was would be in the hall in a minute.

How was Barry feeling? How do you know?

Story 3

The twins loved the old man who lived next door. He used to be an engineer, so he could mend any sort of broken toy. He could fix punctured bicycle wheels, untangle tangled kite strings, work out how to build LEGO® models – Mr Ashworth could do just about anything. He could even make new things out of wood, and had made them both child-sized chairs and painted them lovely bright colours. He never seemed to be too busy to help the twins with their problems. Sometimes Mum said, 'You really can't go and bother Mr Ashworth again.' But Mr Ashworth always said that it was fine: he loved them coming round, and he was glad to help. He was also the one who helped old people with their gardens, pushed stuck cars and cleared the pavements of snow. The twins thought he ought to have a medal.

What sort of man was Mr Ashworth? How do you know?

Story 4

All the boys in Year 5 thought Jeff was wonderful. He was nearly 18, and tall and strong. He sometimes came and helped when they were having PE, or when they played matches against other schools. They knew that Jeff was in the local rugby team, and they had seen videos on his mates' mobiles of Jeff piling into a scrum, getting squashed and jumped on, and coming out muddy and bruised but grinning. They also knew that he was a boxer, and fought people who were nearly pros. Once or twice he had come into school with a black eye, and once a broken arm after rugby. He always just laughed about it and said it was nothing. The younger boys all wanted to be like Jeff.

What sort of boy was Jeff?

Story 5

The Patel family lived in the last of a row of nice, cosy, brightly painted houses, but the very last house in the street wasn't at all like that. It was very old. It hadn't been painted in years, and the woodwork was cracked and crumbling. One of the windows had broken glass in it. The garden was full of weeds. Nobody ever went to the door – when there were any letters, which was not very often, the postman put the letters in a box nailed to the fence. The Patel children had never ever seen the person who lived there. One day, for a dare, they crept into the garden of the old house, and tried to look through a window. While they were crouching there, the front door suddenly flew open, and a terribly tall, thin figure dressed all in black stood there. It was carrying a stick, which it pointed at the children, and in a low, growly voice it said, 'If I catch you, I shall take you to the police station.' Then the figure banged the stick on the ground, and took a step towards the children.

How did the Patel children feel? How do you know?

Story 6

Amy and her friend Diz were playing in the wood at the back of Amy's nan's house. They had found a brilliant tree with branches low enough to climb on. Diz found a little blue eggshell on the path. 'I wonder where the nest is,' she said, looking up. They walked down the path a bit, making sure they could still see Nan's house. Just round the corner there was a little stone hut. 'Ooh, it's like the cottage in Goldilocks and the Three Bears,' giggled Amy. 'Shall we go inside and see if there's any porridge?' said Diz. They pushed the door. It opened easily. Inside there was nothing much: a couple of old plastic garden bags, a spade and a broken bucket. The window was cracked and there were cobwebs everywhere. At the far end was another door. 'We could tidy it up and make it our den,' whispered Amy. Then both girls stopped. There was a faint noise coming from behind the other door. They stared at the door as the handle slowly started to turn.

How did the girls feel? How do you know?

Story 7

On Saturday evening Miss Pink's dance class were doing their end of term show. Bella had been chosen to take the most important part. She was to be the Fairy Queen. She was going to wear a shimmery green and silver dress with real wings attached. She had a magic wand that flashed if she remembered to press the little button on the handle at the right moment. In the afternoon she had been to the hairdressers to have her hair put up in a tight ballerina bun. Mum and Dad and Granny and Grandpa were all coming to watch the show. The girls were starting to get changed now and Miss Pink was fussing around, doing up bows and buttons and mending broken straps. 'Five minutes to go, girls! Do your very best and remember to smile!' Bella heard the music starting. She had to be in position on stage when the curtain went up. She took a deep breath and stepped on to the stage. This was it!

How did Bella feel? How do you know?

Story 8

Mr Crump lived at Number 6 Bell Street. He didn't have a wife or any children, just a black cat called Tibs. Mr Crump loved his garden. He spent hours digging and weeding, clipping and pruning, and he usually won the Best Garden in the Village competition. He grew vegetables, flowers and fruit. Today he was pulling carrots and putting them in a basket to take round to Miss Winnit, who hadn't been very well. He popped a couple of apples into the basket as well, in case he saw the little boys at Number 10. He knew they loved juicy apples straight off the tree. Just then the postman, Ted, appeared. 'Morning, Ted,' called Mr Crump. 'Lovely-looking lettuces you've got there,' said Ted. 'I've got far too many,' replied Mr Crump. 'They all come at once. Here, take a couple,' he said, handing them to Ted. Then he picked up the basket and set off up the road to Miss Winnit's. 'I'll see if she needs any shopping or gardening done while I'm there,' he thought to himself.

What sort of a person is Mr Crump, do you think?

Level 4

Story 1

Ted swallowed hard and took a deep breath when he heard his name called. It was his turn to go on stage and sing.

How was Ted feeling? How do you know?

Story 2

Just at the very last moment Amjit managed to get the ball. One final kick and it was in the goal. The sound of the cheering was deafening as Amjit made his way off the pitch.

How was Amjit feeling? How do you know?

Story 3

Mrs Ragg looked out of the window. Those horrid children next door had kicked their ball into her garden again. She picked up her walking stick and stormed outside, waving it at the two shy little boys peering over the wall.

What sort of person was Mrs Ragg? How do you know?

Story 4

'Anyway, my dad's really rich and my mum drives a sports car, and we always stay in five-star hotels when we go on holiday,' said Tara, standing in the cloakroom with her hands on her hips.

What sort of person was Tara? How do you know?

Story 5

Jed watched his little brother opening his presents. Alf looked really excited when he opened the new LEGO® space set. 'Huh,' muttered Jed. 'It's not that great; anyway, that kind of LEGO® is for little kids. You're just a baby!'

How did Jed feel? How do you know?

Story 6

Kiara was at her Auntie Sue's. Auntie Sue was busy on the computer. She didn't have any children of her own, so there was nothing to play with. On TV there was a programme about people buying houses. Outside it was raining. Kiara sighed. 'How much longer?' she thought.

How did Kiara feel? How do you know?

Story 7

The sky got darker and darker. Soon huge drops of rain began to fall. Nell and her sister looked around for somewhere to shelter, but there wasn't even a tree on the bare hillside. Then Nell heard the first crack of thunder.

How did Nell feel? How do you know?

Story 8

Carlo couldn't believe it. Gordon the guinea pig had been fine that morning when he went to school. And now he was gone. Just a cold little body hunched up in the corner of the cage.

How did Carlo feel? How do you know?

Story 9

Jamilla was looking forward to meeting Layla and Bella at the coffee shop. The others would think she was so cool. She sent Layla a text saying, 'C U there.' The next minute a reply came back, 'Changed plans, not bothering.'

How did Jamilla feel? How do you know?

Story 10

Layla and Bella were at Layla's. Bella said, 'Hey, we're meant to be meeting Jamilla in town; we'd better go.' 'Can't be bothered,' replied Layla. 'But she'll be expecting us,' said Bella. Layla shrugged her shoulders and said, 'So what?'

What kind of person was Layla? How do you know?

Story 11

A ball landed in Mrs Cobb's garden. She stood up, with her hands on her hips, and shouted, 'Don't think you're getting it back. That's the fourth time today and I've had enough!' Then she stomped into the house and slammed the door.

How was Mrs Cobb feeling? How do you know?

Story 12

They were going on holiday to Spain in the morning. Tilly couldn't sleep. What if they were late? What if it was a horrible hotel? What if she didn't like the food? What if she didn't get on with the other kids?

What sort of person was Tilly? How do you know?

Speechmark Ⓢ

Record sheet

Tick the box as each level is achieved

Name _____ **DOB** _____ **Date** _____

TYPE OF INFERENCE	Level 1	Level 2	Level 3	Level 4
ACTION				
PLACE				
OCCUPATION				
OBJECT				
INSTRUMENT				
CATEGORY				
PROBLEM–SOLUTION				
CAUSE–EFFECT				
TIME				
CHARACTER/FEELINGS				

Notes

_____

_____

_____

_____

Continue over

Notes